full
circle
moments

full circle moments

What 20 Years in Neonatology Taught Me About Life, Love & Loss

Terri Lynn Major-Kincade, MD, MPH
The Preemie Doc

publish
your gift

FULL CIRCLE MOMENTS

Published by Publish Your Gift®
An imprint of Purposely Created Publishing Group, LLC

Printed in the United States of America
ISBN: 978-1-64484-542-4 (print)
ISBN: 978-1-64484-543-1 (ebook)

Special discounts are available on bulk quantity purchases by book clubs, associations, and special interest groups. For details email: sales@publishyourgift.com or call (888) 949-6228.
For information log on to www.PublishYourGift.com

Disclaimer: I have tried to recreate events, locales, and conversations from my cherished memories of them. To maintain their anonymity, in some instances, I have intentionally changed the names of family, patients, colleagues, and friends to protect their identities. Many of these recollections represent a composite of several patients and colleagues over the course of my professional journey. Though the time, place, and persons may have been changed, the priceless impact of their influence on my growth as a physician and as a human inspires me every day.

This book is dedicated to the brave babies and families of the NICU (neonatal intensive care unit) who travel unimaginable paths every day and get up to do it over and over again all in the name of hope. To my sister, the first preemie I ever cared for and my inspiration for pursuing neonatology. To my family that shares me often with everyone in my Neonatal world. To my parents who believed I could achieve my dreams. And to God the Author of every beautiful moment in this thing we call life.

Table of Contents

Foreword

Once as part of a Facebook challenge, I was asked to describe my job without revealing my job and I said, "I keep babies in plastic boxes and after several months their parents often thank me for watching them until they were ready to come home." Many people got quite a laugh out of my description, but it's true. Taking care of babies in plastic boxes is a huge part of my job!

Neonatology is a subspecialty of pediatrics that consists of the medical care of newborn infants, especially the ill or premature newborn. It is a hospital-based specialty, and is practiced in neonatal intensive care units, hereafter referred to as NICU. Although I take care of both term and premature infants, most people think of premature infants when one refers to the Neonatal Intensive Care Unit. It is a tribute to the power of media and storytelling that so many people believe that our neonatal intensive care units are filled to the brim with one-pound miracle babies. In actuality the majority of the babies destined to journey to the NICU are in fact late preterm infants, those babies born four to six weeks early at thirty-four to thirty-six weeks gestation and weighing three to four pounds.

In other words, neonatologists are pediatricians who spent several additional years in training to specialize in the care of preterm and sick term infants; pediatricians who only see the babies in the hospital, the tiniest of the tiniest, and the sickest of the sickest. Occasionally they may see former graduates of the NICU in the follow-up clinic for low-birth-weight infants, but usually if you're working in the field of neonatology your primary place of business is the hospital in a magical world of babies where we often meet angels every day.

It's a funny thing to be a neonatologist. Invariably, when someone asks me what I do for a living I hold my breath and try to illuminate my expression when I share that I am a premature baby doctor. Despite the light and pride in my voice, their face always drops a little bit and like clockwork, they say, "Oh my gosh! How can you do that? I just couldn't do it! Doesn't it make you sad?" Their face falls just a little bit more when I share that I specialize in perinatal hospice and neonatal palliative care, yes supporting families whose children may not survive due to severe chromosome problems, birth defects that cannot be fixed, complex surgical conditions, and extreme prematurity. This, my friends, is also about the time they start planning their escape. I can't blame them; how can I explain the wonder of this relatively new world of miracles I get to visit every day? A field that, believe it or not, began at Coney Island in 1896, as an exhibit featuring babies in the very first incubators, or as I like to call them, the plastic boxes! (Blakemore 2018). Advancements in the field during the late 1960s would have a profound impact on my pursuit of a career in modern neonatology.

Certainly, I have seen many babies spend a very short time on this side of heaven, but I've seen many more achieve the impossible and return to tell me about it in their own words and the words of their parents. My job is literally the care of miracles, and my mission is prescribing the Gift of Hope. I truly do believe that I meet angels every day. Some stay but for a moment, others stay longer and come back to visit later. Each moment is sacred, and each face is a chance to be reminded that there is a power greater than ourselves. There is simply no way you can hold a tiny human that fits in your hands and not pause to remember that we are actually living, breathing, and experiencing the miracle of this thing called life.

So how did I come to want to be the type of doctor who took care of the babies in the plastic boxes? Well as I shared earlier, modern neonatology grew in the 1960s shortly after President John F. Kennedy lost his own son to prematurity. Patrick Bouvier Kennedy was born three weeks premature at thirty-seven weeks, weighing four pounds and 10½ ounces. He died at thirty-nine hours of life on August 7, 1963, because of hyaline membrane disease, which is responsible for respiratory distress syndrome in preterm infants. The primary reason for this syndrome is a deficiency of the surfactant protein which is necessary to decrease surface tension in the lungs and allow the lung cells known as alveoli to inflate to and allow for inhalation of oxygen and exhalation of carbon dioxide.

The death of President Kennedy's son at such a good weight and only a few weeks early is said to have been the inciting ember that sparked the medical revolution for the growth of modern neonatology in the United States. Patrick Bouvier Kennedy was life flighted to Boston Children's Hospital and placed in a hyperbaric chamber used for blue babies, traditionally babies with congenital heart problems. Unfortunately, it did not treat hyaline membrane disease. Prior to this event, a physician in Canada had saved a premature baby of similar age and weight as President Kennedy's son using an experimental and controversial new ventilator, but the United States did not have access to the same resources at the time. This traumatic loss for the first family would lead to increased funding for research in neonatal intensive care. Funding by March of Dimes would result in the first exogenous surfactant used to treat hyaline membrane disease as well as the growth of neonatal intensive care units all over the United States (Altman, 2013).

I feel a special attachment to the story of Patrick Bouvier Kennedy, to President Kennedy and his wife Jacqueline in their loss, and the impact their family's tragedy had on the precise field that would become my life's passion. My sister was born in 1968, five years after President Kennedy lost his son to prematurity. She weighed two pounds at birth and was twenty-six to twenty-eight weeks gestation. Over the first few weeks of her life, she would weigh as little as one pound. My parents were told by her doctors that she was very unlikely to survive. Unsure if they were going to ever be able to take her home, they waited three weeks to name her, simply calling her Baby Girl Major. I often wonder about the fear they must have felt, especially since parents had only limited access to visiting neonatal intensive care units at that time, and frequently could only watch their children through the window. But survive and thrive she did, as a result of the availability of surfactant, the availability of ventilators, the improved nutrition for premature babies, and the attention to improved thermo-regulation …yes, those plastic boxes again.

My sister is the first preemie I ever cared for and the inspiration for my desire to become a premature baby doctor. We are only nine months apart and are exactly the same age for three months of the year, but I am still the big sister! I've always loved children and am an innate nurtur-er and empath. I loved playing with my dolls. I loved science. I loved learning. I thought I would either be a pedi-atrician or a kindergarten teacher. As I got older, I learned more and more about my sister's journey as a miracle baby and was fascinated that she had spent part of her life growing in a plastic box. That my parents had watched her grow. That when she came home, she was small enough to sleep in a shoe box. All I could think was, "Wow! How cool is that!??" By the time I started middle school, it was clear that I was going to be a pediatrician. But not just a pediatrician. A pediatrician that takes care of the babies that can fit in your hand. The babies that sleep in the plastic boxes. I later learned that the doctors who took care of the babies in the plastic boxes were called neonatologists. I would also discover that it would take twenty-six years to achieve my dream: twelve years of school, four years of college, four years of medical school, three years of pediatrics and three years of neonatology. Fifteen years after high school. I couldn't wait. The rest, of course, is history!

1

Doctors Who Don't Do Blood

"Life is tough, my darling, but so are you."

STEPHANIE BENNETT HENRY

When your literal job description is to care for babies, you can't help but be excited to go to work. Even though I've been in this field now for over twenty years I still get excited at every delivery. I feel my uterus contracting and pushing with mom. I hold my breath for the cries that we all want to hear in the delivery room. I get nervous about carrying the baby from the operating room table or from the foot of the stirrups once the obstetrician has delivered the baby and hands the baby to the neonatal resuscitation team. Honestly, I always hope that one of my amazing neonatal delivery nurses or equally amazing respiratory therapists will grab the baby and bring the baby to me at the warmer. To this day I'm still afraid that they may slip out of my hands, out of the blanket and onto the floor, swinging by their umbilical cord like a rope. Of course, I've never seen this happen but I'm always worried that it will. On a similar note, can I just say that I hate being in the operating room!

I always laugh when I'm asked how did you know that you wanted to take care of the babies and not the mothers? Do you deliver the babies too? I always shake my head vigorously, "no, I do not," and kudos to my OB friends who, in my opinion, have one of the toughest jobs in the world, the care of mother and baby, at least until I get the baby! I learned pretty early in medical school that I did not like being in the operating room. I didn't like the sterility of it. I always felt like I was in some futuristic location with no control and in many ways, it can be like that because things can change pretty fast in the operating room when someone screams, "Stat C-Section for low heart tones, or worse, no fetal heart tones!"

I hated the smell of blood, and even worse the swoosh of blood as it went through the suction cannister like a red snake. It always looked like gallons to me although many times the surgeon's note would say it was only a few milliliters or cc's depending on your measurement of preference. I passed out a couple of times during my surgery rotation as a medical student. Luckily, I never contaminated the field but my attendings figured out pretty quickly that I was not going into surgery. They invited me to do the post-operative rounds on our surgery patients because that was my thing, talking to and following up with patients, and helping them to navigate their journeys. It was a win-win for both of us. For me, because I no longer had to watch the red river of blood flowing away from patients (I'm sure this river was much bigger in the recesses of my mind than it ever was in real life), and for them because they no longer had to engage in endless conversations with stable post-operative patients.

Incidentally, they did have me evaluated for my constant nose dives in the operating room before revising my rotation. Surprisingly, my very thorough evaluation by an advanced practice nurse (APN) in cardiology revealed that I had a click (extra heart sound) on my heart exam. A subsequent echocardiogram (ultrasound of the heart) revealed that I in fact had mitral valve prolapse (floppy heart valve) and had likely had it my entire life. This was my first introduction to an advanced practice nurse, or nurse practitioner. This is largely related to the fact that APNs became more prominent and started to assume greater responsibilities and autonomy in the early 1990s (Keeling 2015). I sincerely appreciated the time she took to educate me and to make sure that I was in the best shape to complete my medical education. I asked her tons of questions because I had never heard of nurse practitioners, and I wondered if my path might have been different in terms of years of training and dollars in debt had someone shared this career path with me. She broadened my professional world view and for that I am grateful.

I wish I could find my surgery attending today. He recognized my strengths as well as my weaknesses and didn't force me to become something that I was not. That was a huge gift. I passed my surgical rotation in-service exams, but it was with the knowledge that the extent of my surgical adventures would be limited to those necessary for the care and resuscitation of term and preterm infants. I want to thank him and let him know that, to this day, when Dr. Major-Kincade is called to a delivery, she puts on her gown, gloves, and hat, goes straight to the baby warmer, stands in the corner and holds her breath while the Bovie burns for the first cut, blocks out the sound while the blood rushes to through the suction and holds her breath until the baby comes out and one of her favorite neonatal friends brings the baby to the warmer. My job begins when I welcome my new patient into this world. That's a surprisingly good job. So yes! I'm a doctor, but I don't do blood.

2

Embracing Uncertainty: Life on a Tightrope

*"There are only two ways to live your life.
One is as though nothing is a miracle.
The other is as though everything is a miracle."*

ALBERT EINSTEIN

One of the hazards of caring for tiny humans is that invariably you get attached. There are all of the regular baby things like counting ten fingers and ten toes, watching those cute baby smiles even if those who don't believe in magic say it's just gas, and the first yawns and stretches as they discover their power over their bodies outside of their mother's wombs. I've worked in four different states over the past twenty years of my career, and it just never gets old.

One of my favorite parts of this world of babies is hearing the song, usually a lullaby but sometimes the birthday song, once a baby is born. They play it for every baby, not just the healthy babies who are in their parents' rooms, but also the not-so-healthy babies who have to take a trip down the hallway to the neonatal intensive care unit. It's a lovely reminder in the midst of what can often be a hectic day that we are in the presence of miracles; that a new life is pretty freaking special and warrants a sacred moment to attend to the miracle of life happening once again.

There are also some not-so-regular baby things that are a part of life in the neonatal intensive care unit. Watching babies pull out their oxygen tubes repeatedly, seemingly oblivious to the fact that they need the oxygen to stay pink, or maybe they know something we don't! I'm convinced that all the preemies stay up at night and compare notes about how they are going to test their medical providers the next day, and sometimes night, just to keep us on our toes.

I love watching the nurses scold them when they've pulled their feeding tube from their nose (nasogastric tube) or from their mouth (orogastric tube) for the umpteenth time, and l can almost see in the faces of their tiny charges how proud these little humans are of themselves as if to say, "look, I'm a big girl or big boy." The strength of premature babies is nothing short of amazing. The field itself continues to evolve thanks to technology, and it continues to challenge our moral and ethical boundaries.

When I trained in the 1990s, attending a delivery for a baby at less than twenty-four or twenty-five weeks was a pretty big freaking deal. Today, the care of twenty-four and twenty-five weekers seems to be a consistent standard of care across the board in the United States. This brings us to the next frontier, that of twenty-two and twenty-three weekers, which is variable across the United States and even variable within states and cities.

I have no answers here, but I can share that I've cared for several twenty-two- and twenty-three-week infants, many of whom have done well and lived to remind us that neonatology is an imperfect science, and we are still learning. I have also taken care of several who did not do as well and witnessed untold suffering and grief on behalf of patients, parents, and staff. We don't have all the answers, but we owe parents of these infants the answers that we do have.

Early in my career, a father of twenty-three-week twins who had been denied resuscitation, (forcing him and his wife to travel to another facility where their daughters could be given a trial of life), said to me, "Neonatologists are great. We are grateful for the care they provided to our children; however, man does not have the power to look me into the eye and say that my children, my living breathing, human children, are not viable." That has stayed with me and is the one of the reasons I refuse to use the word non-viable when speaking to parents—parents of human children.

Of course, I haven't had the chance to talk to parents of non-human children, but I imagine that my answer would be the same. It is walking this tightrope between what is known and that which is unknown that keeps me fully present and open to the new lessons and new mercies every day that this journey provides. It's really a very precious gift, and I don't take it lightly. There are simply no absolutes. Once you accept that, the rest is not so hard. However, to embrace uncertainty every day of your life—that's pretty damn tough!

3

No Child Left Behind:
Wanting to Adopt Everyone

*"A preemie is a tiny soul that but speaks with the eyes,
kisses with a gaze,
and hugs your heart tighter than you ever
thought possible."*

PEEKABOOICU.NET

In addition to the hazards of becoming attached to the babies that we share with their parents, not all of our babies have parents advocating for them. Those babies can be the toughest to care for because they become everyone's baby, even while child protective services (CPS) is looking for a suitable home other than our mechanical world of beeps, machines, and plastic boxes. This mechanical world is the only home they have ever known.

Anyone who has completed training in pediatrics will be faced with strange phenomena of wanting to care, protect, and nurture those babies who have no home. There are many reasons for this—prior family relationship with CPS, an infant with history of drug exposure requiring long hospital stay, a baby with complex medical problems who the family has decided they are unable to provide the best home, or an abandoned child, just to name a few. In the NICU, the isolation and sometimes abandonment of these babies is painfully obvious. They are the babies no one comes to visit.

My first exposure to a baby like this was during my first year of pediatric residency, my very first month in the neonatal intensive care unit nursery. A very small four-pound baby boy who was born full term but very low birth weight due to exposure to the cytomegalovirus (CMV). CMV is a common virus among most adults in the US, many of whom are not aware that they are even CMV positive. In healthy adults, it can lead to mild upper respiratory infection or no signs and symptoms at all. But if the virus is acquired during pregnancy, it can cause many birth defects including small head, brain calcifications, eye problems, heart problems, and developmental delay. This little boy had been left at a grocery story as part of the baby safe program shortly after birth. I remember meeting him in the NICU and he reminded me of a doll. He had the biggest brightest eyes, but they were set in an older, withered face even though he was just a baby. His microcephaly or smaller head size was very noticeable in comparison to his body, and he reminded me in many ways of a wise, old friend. I loved holding him and feeding him. I wanted him to know that he had taught me a lot. I learned about the process of establishing medical proxy when a child is abandoned. I learned about real life CMV, not just the CMV from my microbiology class or on my immunology exam. He taught me that at the end of the day humans needed humans and I was sure I loved this little guy. I also was convinced at some point that my husband and I needed to adopt him.

Only six months earlier, I had graduated from medical school on a Thursday, got married on Saturday, moved from Los Angeles, California, to Dallas, Texas, and started my pediatric residency that Monday! It is no wonder that my amazing husband thought I had totally lost my mind when I shared that I wanted to adopt the baby from the NICU with CMV. He loved my compassion and my big heart but gently reminded me that we were newlyweds and could not provide this little guy with the life he deserved. More importantly, he reasoned that I would be surrounded by babies my entire career and I couldn't adopt all of them. It was a valuable lesson for me because there would be many more who I would want to take home. I often wonder how my little friend is today. I wish I knew!

Did you know that human babies who develop without human touch have a greater risk of dying? Children who grow up in orphanages actually have a mortality rate of around 30-40 percent. This is perceived to be related to understaffing, resulting in a lack of stimulation for the majority of the babies. Nurturing by parents and caregivers is critical to promote the neurological and psychological development that allows humans to associate touch with pleasure. Similarly, babies who do not experience touch will grow up to fear touch and lack innate feelings of safety usually found in parent-child relationships. These feelings are fundamental in developing the capacity to provide empathy for others (Fagan 2010).

Human touch is a big part of neonatal development and is embraced most obviously in the NICU with kangaroo care. Kangaroo care refers to the practice of holding babies skin to skin, chest to chest on mom or dad (or designated family member) inside the parent's shirt or robe, often under a blanket. Babies who receive kangaroo care maintain their temperature better, regulate their heart rates better, gain weight faster, often go home sooner and are more bonded with parents at the time of discharge (Campbell-Yeo et al. 2015).

When I was a brand-new neonatal fellow (first year of training after residency) there were many mornings after my pre-rounding (examining the patients and checking the vital signs, numbers, and lab results to be ready for my attending) that I would ask the nurses which babies I could hold or which babies I could feed. I couldn't wait to pull out a hospital rocker and hold the babies who had no one to hold them. Often, I would forget that my job was not to be holding the babies, but to be prescribing their medications, their IV fluids, and planning their treatment regimen to make sure they could go home safely. I'm so grateful to the nurses who reminded me that the job of holding, the power of human touch, was equally important to include in my treatment plans.

To this day holding babies is one of my favorite parts of the job. If we are lucky, the hospital has sitters or cuddlers who can care for these babies. A cuddler is a hospital volunteer whose sole job is to cuddle or hold babies. Can you believe that? This has to be the best job in the entire world and a testament to the power of touch. I am confident in my next life I will come back as a cuddler!

4

Riding in the Family Car
When You're Not Family

*"Sometimes the most important thing in a whole day
is the rest we take between two deep breaths."*

ETTY HILLESUM

An inevitable part of my job as a neonatologist is that eventually, I am going to have to deal with death. Unfortunately, it's true not all of my patients will live. This means that since my patients are babies, that I am going to see some babies die. I am going to have to talk to some parents about their babies dying. Sometimes I have this conversation before the babies are even born. Sometimes shortly after birth. Sometimes it's over the phone tearfully asking a family to get to the bedside as soon as possible. Sometimes it's during an active resuscitation, with chest compressions and medications and a child actively trying to leave this realm, with their parents actively and desperately trying to keep them here. Sometimes it's right after surgery. Sometimes it's right before surgery. Sometimes it's even after we've checked everything we possibly could, two or three times, and the child has passed all the required checkpoints to graduate from the NICU, and they still go home, and leave us quietly in their sleep. I've had this conversation many times, but it's never the same because no two children are the same. No two parents are the same, and no two deaths are the same. I look forward to the day when no parent has to say goodbye to their child but until that day, I understand that this is a part of my job. Death is a part of the job of anyone in health care, but sadly, especially for physicians, medical school does not prepare us for this. Residency does not prepare us for this, so we learn by trial and error, modeling our attendings, listening to and observing our patients, and relying on our own life experiences to carry us through each day.

Difficult conversations, end of life patient encounters, managing grief, and compassion fatigue or burnout were not part of my medical school experience. It's unfortunate, but not surprising, that so many physicians are ill-equipped to discuss death and dying. I often do lectures for residents and medical students, and I ask the questions, "Why did you go into medicine? Why do you want to be a physician?" There are so many answers to these questions: to save lives, to help people, because I was sick as a child and doctors helped me, because I lost a loved one and want to give back to the community, or because I love science and the human body, just to name a few. However, no one has ever responded, "I want to go into medicine so I can watch patients die. I want to go into medicine to take care of the dying." Perhaps with the growth of Hospice and Palliative Medicine as a field, eventually this will be an answer, but so far, I have not received this response.

We go into medicine to save lives. That's apparent by the trend of health costs in the United States in comparison to other first-world countries. We are not comfortable with dying and have a lot of work to do with our acceptance of death, medically and culturally. When I was in medical school in the early 1990s, there was no formal training in the art of difficult conversations, discussions including the "D" words of death and dying. I must admit I am kind of jealous that today's generation of medical students, doctors-to-be, residents, and fellows are more likely to receive some didactic training in this area. Often this training is with simulated, standardized patients. That's pretty awesome, especially for our patients. We will not be able to prevent every death, but we can, through our compassion and empathy, do everything possible to provide our patients with a good death, and work hard not to pursue actions that make the experience of death worse.

One of my earliest memories in my medical career of making death worse was attending the funeral of one of my patients. I was very early in my academic career as a neonatal attending and totally in love with my job, my work family, and my patients. I became especially close with the family of one of the very first micro preemies in my care. He ended up with all of the complications to be expected with extreme prematurity. I had a lot of guilt about having been present for his delivery and providing a resuscitation that left him with a life in which he was neurologically devastated. He had spent most of his short life in and out of the hospital. We (I) had asked his parents if they were sure they wanted us to resuscitate him and they had said "yes," but these are impossible choices, impossible scenarios, impossible odds. How can any parent say "no" to the chance that their child might overcome the odds? The burdens of these decisions and the "what ifs" are all too much.

The parents would check in with me from time to time after he went home able to breathe, but not much more, and I would send my prayers and well-wishes. I would not be there when he was admitted to the hospital every several months for lung and brain infections. During one of his admissions, their surgeon asked them if they were sure they wanted to put their baby through another surgery, to which the parents responded, "we do, not but we're not sure if Dr. Major-Kincade will be okay with that."

When my colleague shared their words with me, I cried. Here was a blurring of boundaries. Here was a family desperately trying to do right by their child, to minimize his suffering. To give him more days out of the hospital than in the hospital, however many days that might be. To give him sunshine and light, something he had yet to experience, but they were worried about what I would say. I called them at once and said I supported them. That it had been my pleasure to walk alongside them and their child and that he was blessed to have had them as parents. He went home that day with his parents and had an amazing week being pulled around the city park in his wagon, experiencing the sun, the birds singing, and the sand in between his toes, and he died at home in his parents' arms at the end of that week.

When his family invited me to his funeral, I considered it a rite of passage to attend, to compete the circle of life—the village who had paid witness and homage to his beautiful life, this miracle baby who taught us so much. I walked into the funeral home. I sat in the back pew. I watched the family. I listen to the remarks. At the end of the service, I walked up to that tiny white casket and saw this sweet child and felt my legs buckle. I turned around to the family, hugged the parents, and then fell into the maternal grandmother's arms crying uncontrollably. I was unable to drive to the repast afterwards and was invited to ride in the family car. It was not my finest moment.

I was not family. I had come to support them, but they ended up supporting me. I had even ridden in the family car and left my car at the church. It was a rude awakening for me and a lesson in boundaries and transference.

When I called my clinic admin to see if she could pick me up and take me to the church to get my car, she said, "Dr. Major-Kincade, your job is to support the family. You did not support them today. You took away from their grief. You made their grief worse. If you can't help, then maybe you should not go to funerals." She was right, and that was my last funeral for a very long time. This work is not for the faint of heart. We do grieve with families, but we have not lost our own babies and it is unfair to behave as if we have."

Learning this lesson has made me a better physician. I still occasionally go to funerals, but I leave in my own car.

5

How Are Your Children? Blurring the Lines Between Work and Family

"Some people say they could never work with sick kids, but for me it's the opposite...they have this will to survive that is so strong. They never give up. You can't ask for more than that."

ROSEMARY LIVINGSTON, RN BSN CHILDREN'S
NATIONAL MEDICAL CENTER

When I finally finished my post medical school training (three years of pediatric residency and three years of neonatology fellowship) I could hardly believe it. My dream was finally realized! I was going to be one of the doctors who took care of the babies in the plastic boxes! Babies who were exactly like my sister. I loved every minute of it.

When I shared that I was a preemie baby doctor, people would often say to me, "Oh my gosh! I couldn't do that, you know, take care of sick babies." It no longer bothers me to hear that. I certainly do understand. It can be pretty tough some days, but most days I wouldn't trade it for the world.

During medical school, when my classmates and I were pondering our various professions, it was really clear who was destined to take care of adults and who was destined to take care of babies and children. Of course, there are integrated specialties of Med Peds and Family Practice that allow you to do both, but that's a book for another physician to write. I was always clear that I wanted to take care of babies and children. There is something uncharacteristically pure and unconditionally inspiring to care for a child. One who cannot speak for themselves, but literally wills you to figure out what is hurting or what is not working. To think about the big picture and the minute details, and to fix it all before it's too late. With so many numbers and so many details, the minutia of medicine is why so many clinicians shake their heads and say, "nah, I have to do something else!" A world where every cc counts. Literally, where a drop can make the difference between growth or no growth, fluid overload or no fluid overload, and sedation or no breathing at all.

Our patients in the NICU and of course in the first years of life cannot talk to us. We have to be expert clinicians, and even savvy detectives, to figure out what's going on, and that part never gets old. I really love that part of the field of neonatology, but it's also the part that intimidated many of my friends who chose not to care for babies

and children. Even with all of that, I would not character-
ize neonatology as only the care of babies. For me, it is the
care of babies and families. The babies cannot talk to us,
but the families can, and they do. As we are taking care
of extremely sick, often very small children, we are also
taking care of families. Families that did not sign up for
this. Families for whom no one prepared for this. Every
time I meet a family, I am not only meeting someone who
had no plans to meet me that day, but literally would really rather not have to meet me! And I don't blame them.
The NICU is a world of lost hopes and dreams replaced
by emerging hopes and dreams which often change daily,
if not hourly. It's our job to help our families navigate that
with compassion, honesty, and grace. This is something
most of us did not learn in medical school. However, even
if we did, it wouldn't have provided me with even a quar-
ter of the lessons I have learned from parents along the
way. It is a sacred journey and an immeasurable privilege
to meet these families and partner with them in the care
of their babies. For that, I will be forever grateful. Not only
has this journey made me a better physician, but a better
wife, mother, and human being. It's the gift that keeps on
giving.

So, it is into this sacred space I found myself in 2003,
three years after completing my training and well into my
stride as a brand-new attending physician. It's also the
year my delicate attempts to balance work, life and family

collapsed. As I shared, I loved caring for babies and families. They all became my babies and I truly felt they were family. I loved the science of neonatology, but what I really loved was talking to parents. Empowering them to be advocates for their children. I began to understand that one of my gifts was explaining complex medical conditions and processes to families in a way they could understand and in a way that empowered them to advocate for themselves, ask different questions, and be exposed to different options. I spent a lot of time in family meetings after work, on weekends when I wasn't scheduled to work, and during holidays. My colleagues were happy for my support and my commitment. Unfortunately, no one shared with me that this was a recipe for disaster and a ticket on the express train to burnout!

I was a young mother and wife at the time, married only seven years with two small children, ages three and one. My husband worked in the criminal justice field at the time, and later as a security guard, often working the night shift. I worked long twelve-hour days with thirty-hour shifts every fourth night. During nights when we both were working, our children were in a twenty-four-hour day care. Yes, that's right, a twenty-four-hour day care. Somewhere along the line I lost myself. Between work, clinic, and being everything to all of my families, there was very little of me left for my husband and my children. My own children didn't really know me, and when I would go to pick them up from daycare, the teachers often acted surprised. One even commented, "Oh, I thought their dad was a single parent!"

One particularly "aha moment," as Oprah would say, happened as I was walking through the neonatal ICU nursery one day and one of my favorite nurses said, "Hi Dr. Kincade! How are the children?" To which I responded, "Who, Baby Williams? Baby Jones? Baby Smith? Baby Gonzalez?" Quickly rattling off just a few of the children I needed to see that day. She paused for a moment and just looked at me. Then she repeated herself, "No, Dr. Kincade. How are *your children*? You know, Stevi and Terrence?" I was mortified that in that moment I had listed the names of my patients instead of my own children, and I knew something would have to change.

At the time, academia did not afford me the flexibility that I needed and wanted to be a mother, a wife, and a neonatologist. This was compounded by the fact that my mentor was a senior white male, much like many of my other mentors, whose wife had been a stay-at-home mother. The other women in our department were not married, or did not have partners or children, so I had no role models for how to do this better, but I knew that what I was doing was not going to work. Therefore, it's no surprise that four years into academic medicine, and one year after winning the physician of the year award, I made one of the scariest and bravest decisions of my career and life.

I decided to leave academic medicine for private practice. I chose my family and trusted that the right job would find me. I was blessed to be able to join a wonderful practice that allowed me to work primarily weekend nights. It allowed me to be home Monday through Thursday. I worked Friday, Saturday, and Sunday nights, but was able to be home in the mornings after my shifts and attend church, soccer and football games, track meets, and movie matinees.

My children were able to come to the hospital with me during the evenings. They took swimming lessons twice a week. I joined the Parent Teachers Association (PTA) and became the head copy room mom. It was an amazing volunteer position which allowed me to coordinate all the other mom volunteers on a weekly basis to complete copy requests from the teachers for their classroom activities. It was so much fun! We had family dinners, amazing vacations and super cool games of hide-and-seek followed by bedtime stories. I was able to do that through most of their elementary years until middle school. I love the life that my husband and I have built with our children. But most of all, I learned that it is possible to be a great clinician, to have wonderful relationships with your patients, and at the same time, to be a happy wife, mother, and person outside of the hospital. I am not sure I would have learned or believed that had I stayed in academic medicine.

Boundaries. Boundaries. Boundaries. My career has taught me the value of boundaries, and I'm grateful for that. Women working in medicine today navigate multiple roles, juggle competing priorities, and discover that there are so many options. Boundaries matter. For me, the best test has been that today, when someone asks me how my children are doing, I am clear that they are talking about *my own children*. They'll be clear too since I love talking about my own children. I have an amazing son pursuing his bachelor's degree in media and animation, and an amazing daughter currently navigating her third year of veterinary school. I still think their dad is their favorite, but I am a very close second. And for that I'm grateful.

6

When Professional and Personal Dreams Collide: Nightmares Can Happen

"Your work is going to fill a large part of your life, and the only way to be truly satisfied is to do what you believe is great work. And the only way to do great work is to love what you do. If you haven't found it yet, keep looking. Don't settle. As with all matters of the heart, you'll know when you find it."

STEVE JOBS

This chapter was previously published in *Chicken Soup for the Soul: Power Moms Series*. I am reiterating it here because it contains a more detailed explanation of several of the events and instances that I previously mentioned. For as long as I can remember, I have wanted to be a pediatrician. Not just any pediatrician, but the kind that took care of the tiny babies in the plastic boxes. My sister had been premature. I was fascinated by the fact that she lived for three months in a plastic box while my parents watched her grow, and then one day she came home. Eventually, I did realize my dream and learned that the pediatrician who took care of the tiniest babies was called a neonatologist.

Every time I walked into the neonatal unit I felt such pride—I loved the families and their precious babies. I loved being the one they leaned on, trusted, prayed with, and cried with—and most of all I loved being the one who finally got to send their baby home. Somewhere along the line, I started loving that too much. I started loving the role and the image more than I cherished the service. I slowly began to believe I was indispensable, and I made decisions that negatively impacted my own family.

In the fall of 2001, I began caring for a baby with many problems related to an abnormally developed intestine. He spent nine months in the hospital. The more I cared for him and his family, the more I resisted allowing other doctors to care for him. I began to work weekends I wasn't scheduled to work—deciding to leave my husband and two children early in the mornings while they still slept—and then rushing back to spend some time with them before I returned to work the next morning. Mornings I wasn't scheduled to work, I begged to work, and my co-workers were more than willing to let me work so they could enjoy time with their families. My husband began to pick the kids up from daycare while I stayed longer hours at the hospital making sure my patient was stable and his family's needs were met. I was off for Thanksgiving but opted to stay in town so I could look in on my patient just in case—my husband obliged.

In a passing instant I noticed how different my husband looked to me—I wondered when he decided to grow a full beard and was too embarrassed to ask how long it had been there. I noticed a new tattoo on his back of an angel with the names of our children written on each of his wings. How in the world had I missed that? I also noticed how clingy the kids were to him when we went out as a family. I felt like an outsider. I wanted to talk to him about all these things, but I was too busy to process it, too busy to give myself a chance to feel anything more than brief concern.

Then came Christmas—I was scheduled to be off again, but Jared required another surgery. He was nine months old now and smiled when I came into the room. How could I leave him for Christmas? How could I leave his family? I decided to work Christmas. I don't remember Christmas that year with my husband or kids. I should; my daughter was four and my son was two—the perfect ages to really appreciate the magic. I vaguely remember a rocking horse—and a jumping Tigger. What I remember most is carrying Jared around the hospital on Christmas Day with a Santa hat on. People asked me how my kids were,

"Baby Jones, Baby Williams? Baby Lopez?"
"No—your two at home, Stevi and Terrence."

What was I doing, spending all my time working at the hospital? I reminded myself I was performing a great service, and how much the families appreciated and needed me. In January of 2002, I was called to an impromptu meeting in the Nursing Lounge—annoyed at being pulled away from my patients, I went reluctantly. I found a room full of people with balloons, confetti, and well wishes. I was the hospital physician of the year—they noted that I was the first African American, and the youngest to receive the award. I felt elated. I thought of all those childhood dreams, fulfilled in that moment—I thought of how proud my parents would be.

During the ceremony I anxiously waited for the CEO to read my bio. His words chilled me to the core and I remember each one to this very day, "Dr. Kincade is loved by all of the nursing staff and extremely dedicated. She routinely works weekends that she is not scheduled to work. She stays after work even after checking out, and this year she worked Thanksgiving and Christmas vacation to be with a complicated patient when she could have taken the time to be off her family. She chose to give up her holiday to care for our patients."

I cried. I felt sad at all the missed opportunities to be with my husband and to nurture my children. I felt completely offended by this person who gave up Thanksgiving and Christmas to work when she could have been with her family, the person who had raved about finding twenty-four-hour daycare so she could stay later at work. I struggled to swallow the lump in my throat. I thought instead of getting physician of the year, how badly I wanted to be wife and mother of the year.

As I walked slowly to the podium to get my plaque, with tears streaming down my face, I forced a smile to take my picture with the CEO. I promised myself to leave this environment and work where people didn't think it was a good thing to give up Thanksgiving and Christmas unless you had to. I wanted to join the PTA. I wanted to play games with my husband and children—I wanted to know the real answer to "How are your kids?" and I wanted the teachers to know who I was when I picked up the children. I wanted to breathe again and believe that somewhere I could be a mommy, a wife, and a doctor. And that's exactly what I did.

Eighteen years ago, I left the university. I received much criticism, as everyone lamented how I threw my career away. I traded that career for a better career, because now I am a Power Mom. I smile as I drop the kids off at school and return in the afternoon to be first in the carpool lane. I laugh at how loud I am screaming at the soccer and basketball games. I dance with the kids at the Valentine's party as they all cheer for the cool mom. I get tears in my eyes when my daughter shares how much it means to her that I came on the field trip. I finally got my dream to be on the PTA and pinch myself because I am so excited to be on a committee. "Can it get any better?"

When someone asks me after a long and hot field day, "How do you have time to be so active, do you work?"

"Yes, I do, I'm a neonatologist."

"No way. How can you be a doctor and be so active at school?"

My smile grows into a grin, "I only work weekend nights, for three weekends a month. I have Monday, Tuesday, Wednesday, and Thursdays completely off." I can hardly contain my joy as I remember something said to me at the beginning of medical school. "You can have it all; you just can't have it all at the same time." And I think, oh yes you can. You truly can. When you listen to your spirit, sometimes you realize that what you once thought was all and what for you now is all may no longer be the same thing. Your new all may not be that far from your reach. But you have to take the first step. Sometimes that means leaving behind one big award for a million daily awards. What will *your* award be?

7

When Babies Cry, Please Don't Write for Codeine

"It's a great day to save lives."

DR. DEREK SHEPHERD, *GREY'S ANATOMY*

I could probably write two or three more books about the things nurses have taught me during my career and the lessons I have learned from babies. One of the earliest lessons was to always get up and go see the patient when you are on call. Being tired does not matter. When the nurse calls, get up and go see the patient, that's lesson number one. Lesson number two, when the nurse says she is concerned, get up and go see the patient. For most of my career, I have been surrounded by nurses who have tons of experience and who have been in the medical field longer than I have. For me, that's very valuable, and I look at every interaction as an opportunity to learn. Now that I am twenty-plus years into my career, I frequently encounter nurses recently out of training and love the opportunity to partner, collaborate, and develop care plans together. After all, they are at the bedside for twelve hours. I may be on call twenty-four hours, but I am not at one bedside for twelve hours continuously, so I need and very much appreciate the insight of my nursing colleagues.

Early in my career, as I was learning how to actually be on call, not be tired, stay focused, and manage multiple patients, I had some challenges, as many young interns do, with keeping up and wanting to do the best job. I remember one particularly stressful call night as if it was yesterday. I had already been up for eighteen hours straight with no breaks, no dinner, no naps, just a bathroom break and the usual intern call special graham crackers, peanut butter, and apple juice. I was on the general pediatrics rotation during the winter. I had already helped to admit five babies from the emergency room, all sick with respiratory infections, croup, flu, and many with reactive airway disease or bronchiolitis and wheezing like asthma. I had also admitted a couple of sickle cell patients with pain and respiratory infections.

Between midnight and three am, a patient came in with vomiting and diarrhea. She was less than one year of age and admitted for dehydration. During the night, the baby had intermittent crying felt to be related to crampy abdominal pain. Her nurse called to say that the baby was crying. I was new to pediatrics, tired, and in-between two really sick respiratory patients. My first thought was, "Okay. Babies cry." She shared that she thought the baby was in some pain. I gave a verbal order for Tylenol with codeine (yes, we were still using Tylenol with codeine at the time). I then went to see another patient and called back to check on the patient. The nurse shared the baby was better but had a red-tinged stool. I hung up the phone and ran to see the baby. I remembered crampy abdominal pain, red-tinged stool, and hoped that she didn't have a sausage-shaped mass that I could feel in her abdomen. Because that would mean intussusception.

Intussusception is a fancy term for when the intestine goes inside itself. It is a surgical emergency. I found my patient sleeping soundly in her bed and indeed felt a sausage-shaped mass inside of her abdomen. I notified my senior resident and literally ran down with the patient and the nurse to radiology, where they were waiting to do an emergency air enema to relieve the bowel from being inside itself. During the procedure, her intestine perforated (developed a small hole), which caused her abdomen to become very big from extra air. Surgery came immediately and took her to the operating room where she was repaired and went home a couple of weeks later, totally normal.

The case was later presented during our case reviews, and I was applauded as an intern for diagnosing intussusception. I made a point to highlight the nurse who first recognized crying, crampy pain that was not colic. I also made a point to say that Tylenol with codeine will no longer be my first thought for crying babies. I never wrote for it again, and today, you can't write for it at all. It's been almost twenty-two years since that case, but I think about that baby every time I hear that a baby is crying. It was also the first time I actually had a patient who looked exactly like all the questions I had studied for on my pediatric practice exams. To this day, there are two things that I always do. Always thank the nurse for calling, and always go and see the patient before writing for anything. This has served me well for over twenty years. It's a good mantra for many life circumstances. Listen to the concern. Evaluate the situation before acting. I'd say that's golden. Wouldn't you?

8

Come Right Now: Your Baby is Dying

*"The expectation that we can be immersed in suffering
and loss daily and not be touched by it
is as unrealistic as expecting to be able to walk
through water without getting wet."*

NAOMI RACHEL REMEN

I've tried really hard to paint a rosy picture of the joy that I feel caring for babies and families in the almost foreign and isolated world of the NICU. But let's face it! My job is, in fact, the care of critically ill infants, some of whom might not survive despite our best efforts. Even after twenty-plus years in the field and seeing many babies not survive their illness or their extreme prematurity, I am always still extremely sad, and at times even a bit taken aback. I know the odds. I know the reality. I know the signs and symptoms of likely impending death but that doesn't mean that I'm not hoping, willing, and daring right along with the parents to see and achieve the impossible.

Sometimes the impossible looks very different than what we imagined—the impossible is just the peace and acceptance of a chance to experience the sacred gift of the life of another human being, no matter how short. It's taken me a long time to understand this, and honestly, I still struggle quite a bit. I get my strength from babies, from parents, and of course, from God. I remind myself that we are created in His image every time I see a sweet baby's little face.

I remember the loss of every baby as if it were yesterday. I can see the families' faces, the tears in their eyes, the fear behind their eyes, and the voices that want to say so much but are currently mute, silenced with the heaviness of an unbearable loss. I remember the nurses calling me with updates on unexpected clinical changes, and the lump in my own throat, as I know at this point in my career what these changes mean.

Babies in the neonatal intensive care unit nursery can die for several reasons, but some of the most common reasons include severe infections (some of which they are born with, others that they may acquire or develop after being in the NICU or out in the world with very fragile immune systems); birth defects that we cannot fix like heart problems or severe chromosome problems; extreme prematurity with lungs that we cannot inflate or provide enough oxygen in spite of our powerful machines; severe bleeding in the brain that changes the ability to breathe spontaneously or walk, talk or have interactions with family; severe stomach infections that require surgery; or challenges at delivery or just before delivery that affect the babies' heart rates in a way that they are unable to recover. Each one of these situations is unimaginable for families and health care providers and the definition of our worst nightmare. But for us it's a day, a moment. For our families, it's a lifetime of an altered expectation.

There's really no way I can offer this moment, the experience, or the process justice on these pages. But I want to hold space to honor all the babies we've loved and lost. The ones for whom we tried but for whom technology was not enough, those born too soon but who remain here still in our hearts and minds long after their bodies are gone. For the many parents to whom I've had to say way too many times, "Come now...your baby is dying," I'm so very sorry for your loss!

I remember the mom and dad who were downstairs at the gift shop purchasing clothes to take their daughter home when her heart rate suddenly dropped out of the blue and she required cardiopulmonary resuscitation (CPR). A baby who was supposed to go home the next day after four long months in the NICU. I remember having to run downstairs to the gift shop, interrupting their purchases of hospital souvenirs and teddy bears to say, come now, your daughter dropped her heart rate and is getting CPR. I remember them saying, "What?!" and me finally breaking saying, "Please come now…your daughter is dying." I remember running back with them to the NICU and finding their sweet baby no longer pink but blue. No longer smiling but lifeless, still receiving CPR after fifteen minutes with no response. I remember his mom pushing everyone out of the way and saying, "Just stop. Stop right now. Give me my baby." And so, we did.

It's been more than twenty years since that happened and I still remember it like it happened yesterday. It was not the first death I experienced in the NICU, but it was one of the first that taught me a very pivotal lesson. When we say that babies are okay, that is relative. They are okay for this moment. They are okay for this moment. Things change very quickly in the NICU. Unpredictably quickly. It's a very peculiar kind of limbo in which we live. A borrowed space of time, life, and biology, doing the work of the womb and hoping we get it right. Hoping everything works out okay. Most of the time it does, but many times it does not. It's why we both jokingly and somberly say, "never trust a preemie," and sadly, we mean it. They are truly the most amazing and the most frightening creatures on Earth, and I have a very healthy respect for them!

9

Sometimes It's a Circus: The Blessings and Burdens of Walking the Tightrope of Viability

"This is not general surgery on a miniature scale. These are the tiny humans. These are children. They believe in magic. They play pretend. There is fairy dust in their IV bags. They hope, and they cross their fingers, and they make wishes, and that makes them more resilient than adults. They recover faster, survive worse. They believe."

ARIZONA, *GREY'S ANATOMY*

Normally when I say to someone that I'm a neonatologist they look at me with a blank stare, unless of course they have had a premature baby or a very sick term baby. I usually follow the sentence, "I'm a neonatologist" with the words, "I'm a pediatrician who cares for premature babies, you know—the ones who can fit in the palms of your hands or the term babies who are very sick and may require surgery." I can literally bet my entire life savings (which isn't much) on the next words to leave their lips. "Wow, how sad. I couldn't do that. God Bless you."

It always gives me great pause when I hear those words. I don't think of my job as sad at all. I consider it a great blessing and a huge privilege to hold the hands of those parents who have a baby that must be admitted to a neonatal intensive care nursery. I get to see a miracle every day and often I meet angels. It's a place so few will ever visit, and it's so much bigger than the miracle babies that you see on television. As I mentioned previously, I've wanted to be a neonatologist, aka preemie doctor, since I was a very little girl and realized that my sister had been premature. That she was small enough to fit in the palm of your hands. That she spent her first months of life in a plastic box known as an incubator. And that the doctors who cared for those babies were called neonatologists, and the rest, as they say, is history.

But neonatology is a relatively new branch of pediatrics; I am constantly amazed at the ultramodern field today and a tad bit frightened. We are saving babies today that we were not able to save fifteen or twenty years ago, babies that during my training we did not have the equipment to offer a so-called "trial of life." In the late 1960s, the field of neonatology was just beginning. My sister was born in 1968. She was a micro preemie, born at twenty-six weeks gestation and, at one point, weighing only one pound. This was just five years after President Kennedy had lost his son to prematurity—a son who was four pounds, ten ounces, and born at thirty-seven weeks, or almost three weeks early. Unfortunately, he was born when neonatal intensive care nurseries were just beginning and, despite a heroic transport, he could not be saved. I carry both of their legacies with me every time I enter a delivery room, and every time I hold a tiny human in my hand. The feeling leaves me mystified even now, twenty years into my career.

This issue of the viability of a human life has grown because technology has gotten pretty good at saving little humans, but at what cost? We now have the capacity, in many cases, to offer a trial of resuscitation to twenty-two-week infants—infants almost four and a half months early—most of whom who do not survive, and some who survive, but with significant neurologic handicap. It's a slippery slope and a very perilous tightrope, and I have no idea what the right answer is, and I dare say that no neonatologist does. This push has largely been in response to parental desires, and in my opinion, very understandable. I don't know the right answer for every family, but I do know I'm in this profession for a reason. I try to support the life that's presented to me for the time that the life is here. Sometimes the support is warmth, human touch, soft words, a prayer; other times the support is machines, tubes, wires, and more prayers…sometimes you just don't know.

About a year ago, I was forced to walk that tightrope, and the power of the human spirit wrapped in one little one-pound body has continued to both haunt and encourage me. I started my shift, like so many shifts, hearing a report about how many sick babies were in the ICU nursery and how many more sick babies were coming. I was told about a baby whose mother desperately wanted her to survive, but unfortunately the mother had gone into preterm labor at only twenty-two weeks. At this hospital, and many hospitals, fetuses who are less than twenty-three weeks are considered to be non-viable. On a personal note, I hate the word non-viable and never say it when speaking to families unless they use the word themselves in reference to their pregnancy. But what does that mean? It means that despite heroic measures, the infant is more likely to not survive than survive, and that if the infant does survive, he or she would do so very likely with grave handicap.

To intervene in this scenario is often perceived as cruel to the infant. This mother was going to be twenty-three weeks at midnight. The current time was 7 p.m. What a choice. It's actually no choice at all. If the baby were to be born before midnight, we would not intervene but provide comfort care. If the baby were to be born after midnight, we would try to resuscitate the baby. Again, this is no choice. This is the tightrope that I hate. This is the slippery slope that has you questioning your life choices in a matter of seconds. When I spoke with the mother, she shared she understood the risk, but what she really wanted to know was that, if her child was born before midnight and she held her child until midnight, would I come then and try to resuscitate the baby if the baby was still alive. She cried. I cried. We both prayed that her child would not be born before midnight, but her labor was progressing and the child was indeed coming. I really hated those arbitrary lines around viability. I remember every baby I've left and so many more that I tried to save, and they all leave me wishing that no one ever went into preterm labor. It is the epitome of being between a rock and a hard place…no easy answers.

The child was delivered in bed at exactly 11:30 p.m., thirty minutes before the arbitrary cut off time for the coveted trial of life. And guess what? The child was actively crying—and moving. Surprisingly, a twenty-two-week infant crying, moving, daring me to leave her in her mother's room. What to do? Leave? Stay? Do no harm? But life in the NICU is unfortunately filled with harm in the name of saving lives. Some babies will recover from this harm, but not all of them. I picked the baby up and brought her to the warmer. She was giving it her all and the minutes were ticking. I knew the mom understood that her life could very well include blindness, cerebral palsy, and handicap, but so could any other life.

So, we proceeded with a trial of life, which included placement of a breathing tube, oxygen therapy, and a respirator. Her first several days were very rocky and she was very unstable. Her mother made her DNR (do not resuscitate), but her heart never stopped. Her lungs got stronger. She got stronger. She never had another rough day after two weeks of age. She went home without any equipment. With no brain injury, no eye injury, and actually breastfeeding. In twenty years, I had never seen that, and I don't know if I will ever see it again, but I am blessed to have witnessed a rare miracle. A rare moment where the art of medicine superseded the science of medicine and one little human spirit literally dared me to leave her in the delivery room.

10

A Pediatrician Struggles with Her Own Advice: Do as I Say, Not as I Do

"Then one day when you least expect it, the great adventure finds you."

EWAN MCGREGOR

I've been told that for those who foresee a career in medicine, few aspiring healers actually go on to choose the specialty that they originally envisioned for themselves. This chapter was originally published in *Medium and Doximity Op Med,* but it is important to me that I share it with you at this time. I've known since I was five years old that I wanted to take care of children, as documented in my kindergarten "All About Me" book. I clearly proclaim in the book's crayon-written foreword that I had plans to become a kindergarten teacher or a baby doctor. As I became older, I was fascinated by the idea that my sister was premature and that, when she was born, she was small enough to fit into the palm of your hand; she had spent her early months in a plastic box.

Eventually, I learned that the baby doctors who took care of the babies in the plastic boxes or incubators were called pediatricians. Then I was excited to learn that they were in fact, pediatricians who specialized in the field of neonatal-perinatal medicine, neonatologists for short, and my fate was sealed. I was going to be a neonatologist. Along the way, I mentored kids, participated in story time at the library, played doctor with my dolls, and volunteered in the nursery. During medical school, I researched childhood developmental patterns, developed parental resources to ameliorate stress, worked at the Centers for Disease Control and Prevention (CDC) and studied the effects of childhood lead poisoning. During residency, I realized that although I loved the NICU, I really loved follow-up of NICU babies and was blessed to run the follow-up clinic for several years. Is there anything better than empowering a parent to realize that they can truly parent; that they are capable of being everything their child needs?! I think not. It's the best feeling in the world, and I consider myself a parent advocate first and a pediatrician second.

But then I had my own children and realized a couple of things.

I had my first child during my neonatology fellowship. As a new mother, I enjoyed every other night call at Parkland Hospital, which at the time boasted one of the busiest delivery services in the United States. My hubby and I tag-teamed and did the best we could, but it was hard, even with our resources. I realized that although I had encouraged many moms that breast is best, I was unable to maintain my milk supply during my training as a fellow; I had to stop at six months. I realized that, although I shared with my families that their babies should sleep on their backs and not their tummies, my baby preferred her tummy. My baby had colic. My baby was very gassy, and it was a bit challenging to let her cry it out. How many mothers had I encouraged to let the baby cry it out? It was also a bit challenging to walk around all night rocking her. Sleep deprivation became my norm. I knew she wasn't supposed to sleep in our bed, but she found herself in our bed more often than not. I wasn't proud of this. I knew she wasn't supposed to have her pacifier beyond the first year, but I also knew that there were some battles I didn't have the energy to fight. So, yes, she had it until pre-K. Today, at almost twenty-four, she has perfect teeth and never required braces.

I remember feeling like a hypocrite. Being calm, reassuring and telling parents that their feelings were normal. That they would manage their routine. That yes mommy should just keep pumping. That yes, the baby should always stay on his or her back. That yes, they should hasten to get rid of the pacifier before it's too late and if possible don't even start! This was of course before the sudden infant death syndrome (SIDS) data in support of pacifier use (Moon et al. 2012). I struggled with advising parents during the day and barely meeting those anticipatory guidelines during the night. I was in fact Super Doc with all the answers during the day and exhausted mommy doing my best to keep up at as soon as my workday ended. Hubby and I often smile now, that our daughter was such a good baby while we were trying to figure out how to be parents, and be husband and wife, and manage our career and household.

Two years later, in my last year of fellowship, we were blessed to have our second child, a boy. I was an attending physician now. We had more resources. Hubby and I had figured out how to make it work, and we did. But what if we hadn't? What of those parents who are still trying to figure it out? What if you do have to make some concessions along the way? How can we more realistically support parents? Where are the Ages and Stages that meet families in the middle? We cannot support children without supporting parents.

Fast-forward twenty-seven years. Our kids are now twenty-four and twenty-one, and appear to be doing well. I have over twenty years of experience under my belt. I have taken and renewed my Neonatal and Pediatric Boards twice. I keep up with the literature. I am keenly aware of the Ages and Stages Guidelines, but I have never forgotten what a desperate time new parenthood was for us! We recently kept our great nieces for a week and continue to do so each summer. At the start of this annual tradition, they were ages eighteen months and four years, for one week. What a reality check! Again, I learned a lot.

I had forgotten how much energy is required to keep up with a toddler and a preschooler. As I relearned from my nieces, after a full day either in the home or out of the home, you might find yourself violating the screen time guidelines a time or two. Because you need a moment. Because dinner has to be prepared. Because life. And we can't beat up parents about that.

And let's not forget about the guidelines for routines. Routines are so important for children. We tried with our nieces. We tried to have a set dinner time, a set breakfast time, a set lunch time. We tried to limit screen time. We tried to have a set bath time. We tried to have a set bed-time. Oh, and we tried to put them in their own beds as well. This was at best a work in progress and at worst a disaster!

Sometimes they were in bed by nine, but most of the time they were not! Bath time was great fun, but never at the same time. Story time was a huge hit, but never at the same time. Even bedtime often violated screen time, as movies were quickly revealed to be the way we all went to sleep. But what about reading? Reading is fundamen-tal, I wholeheartedly agree! Did we read books? Yes, we read books; the kids loved them. But, after several books, we watched Beauty and the Beast (their favorite) over and over and over. I felt like I received a pediatrics parenting demerit each time!

Lastly, meals. Yes, children should have fresh vegetables. No sugary sweets. Healthy alternatives. I agree! I say it every day to my patients. But to provide healthy alternatives to your children, you must be providing healthy alternatives to yourself. We learned that we eat out a lot. We had to force ourselves to make sure the girls were getting healthy alternatives, and they loved those alternatives, often saying, "Yay, real food tonight." But this was a hard adjustment for us, even with our resources and twenty years of parenting experience. Of course, we thoroughly enjoyed our time with our great nieces, but I wondered what do young families do who are overwhelmed? Families who need resources and easy alternatives? What about single parents? How much anticipatory guidance have I given to families who are overwhelmed, who are stressed, who are doing the best they can, but even their best doesn't meet the guidelines for best parenting practices?

I will of course continue to encourage and endorse the American Academy of Pediatrics (AAP) guidelines for effective parenting and positive child development. But I will also remember to ask mom or dad how they are doing. Sometimes the best guidance is "It's okay." It really is okay. Exhale…and try again tomorrow. And then I tell myself the same thing. It will be a year before we keep our great nieces again. They will be two and five. This time, we will be ready!

11

Miracles in the NICU: Awareness Season

"You never know how strong you are until being strong is your only choice."

BOB MARLEY

September, October, and November are my favorite months of the year because I get to talk about several issues close to my heart across all my social media platforms, and my friends, family, and colleagues give me a pass. A pass to share the wonder, mystery, and sometimes stark horrors that make up this often-hidden world of caring for babies and families. Of course, I talk about these issues daily anyway, but when I add the Awareness Month, they let me talk just a little bit longer!

September is National Infant Mortality Awareness Month, a time when we all pause to reflect on the thousands of babies who die each year before their first birthday and the causes of those deaths including prematurity, birth defects, and sudden infant death syndrome. Recently, it was also designated as neonatal intensive care awareness month. The goals for Neonatal Intensive Care Awareness are not only to bring attention to those medical conditions requiring admission to the NICU but also to the staff who care for those babies and the awesome families who celebrate these tiny fighters. October is Pregnancy Loss and Infant Death Awareness Month, which focuses more on the silent pain of miscarriage, still birth, and early infant deaths. One in four women is impacted by pregnancy loss which means it's more common than many realize and likely has impacted this reader or someone they know or work with. Just think about that. One in four represents a lot of families. It's numbers like this that give me such great pause. November represents Prematurity Awareness month and rounds out the story that begins with a reminder that not all babies survive, that not all babies are born healthy, that not all pregnancies end with a live birth, and that one in seven babies begin their lives with an incredibly challenging journey through the Neonatal ICU.

Although I am constantly walking the line between life and death, between beginnings and oh-so-short endings, I am constantly blessed in ways that can't be measured in words. What have I learned in these moments between life and death, beginnings, and endings, from these tiny warriors and the people they call family? On the path called awareness, the journey forces the traveler to accept that pregnancy loss is real, that infant loss is real, and that the neonatal intensive care unit is an amazing and scary place, and that prematurity is the biggest contributor to infant mortality today.

I have learned that angels come in many sizes shapes and packages. They may hold my hand at the bedside when I am trying not to cry in front of a parent. They may visit in a sweet prayer circle as we stand around the tiny bed of an even tinier soul. They may arrive bringing pizza during a horrible night shift when no one has had time to eat or even go to the bathroom for twelve hours. They may visit for few moments in the delivery room, just to allow us to witness a few precious breaths or the occasional fragile heartbeat, and to remind us of our humanity. As if anyone in this business could ever take for granted the fragility of life. But then things go back to normal and angels come back to visit, this time for days, even months in the NICU, and then decide suddenly without warning but with great fanfare, that their work here is done. In the quiet. Through the tears we receive again. Another reminder that none of us are in control. Yes, here more than ever we do understand that control is an illusion!

I have learned that miracles are not trapped in the pages of my bible, but miracles are living, breathing, crying, and walking around me every day. I just have to open my eyes, clear my ears, and take time to breathe. So, I open my eyes and clear my ears and I see a baby crying, kicking, and screaming—and I smile. Why? Because it's a baby I thought would not be here. Yep, miracle. I see a baby final-ly get to go home after ten long months…months when so many of us had given up. Yep, miracle. I see a family visit yearly to celebrate the staff and honor the memory of their child—a sweet angel gone too soon—and I see staff comforted. Who does that? Yep, miracle. I see foundations started in memory of babies gone…and in hope of babies to come. Yep, miracle. And I see me a little brown girl from Louisiana blessed with being able to live her dream in a world where many are not. Yep, miracle.

The little people have taught me to *live* in the mo-ments—the moments in *between* life and death, in *between* beginnings and endings, for in this great big thing we call life, that's truly all we have. And you know what the Angels are there. The miracles are there. It's enough for the little people. It's enough for me? I pray that it's enough for you too!

12

Numbers are Numbers but Life Is Life: Just Breathe

"Nobody but Nobody is going to stop breathing on me."

DR. VIRGINIA APGAR

Fortunately, in the NICU there is always something new to learn and a new miracle to behold. I'd like to share with you what I have learned from NICU parents about strength. I am often amazed at the strength of the parents of our tiniest babies, the fighters, the one-pound heroes and sheroes that are often celebrated in the media. What goes through their minds as one physician after another begins to share grim and frightening statistics shortly after birth? At a time when parents should be contemplating when the baby shower will be, which crib is best, and what color the nursery should be, doctors are saying, "Your child has only a 30-40 percent chance of living," or, "if your child does live, he or she may have severe brain damage or may be blind or may develop intestinal or cardiac complications." That's a lot to throw at a family, and then we have the audacity to add, "We will do everything we can, but it does not look good." How do they keep smiling through the tears? How do they persevere to the silver lining? In twenty years, I have yet to find the complete answer to this question. But just recently I got a bit of a glimpse through a 410-gram (fourteen-ounce) human being.

He was only the second smallest baby I had ever taken care of that lived, and boy was he a teeny tiny thing. I looked at him, he looked at me, both of us wondering what on Earth was going on. He was there when I shared those grim numbers with her parents, but like them, he kept on breathing. Like them, he kept on kicking. Like them he kept on showing up saying,

"What's next, Dr. Kincade? What's next?" I am breathing.

My heart is beating. Your move!"

In one of those rare moments of me, the Giant, staring at him, the not so giant, he seemed to say, "Kincade… I heard what you said… but you know what? Numbers are just numbers… but life is life... and I'm here, so keep it moving! What else are you going to do? Keep staring at me every day singing the same ole song? I am ready for a new tune!" And a new tune is what he got. No one likes to hear the same ole song over and over and over again—unless it's Prince—I kind of like hearing him on repeat!

It's been almost eight years since I stared into the eyes of that fourteen-ounce human and now he's a whopping fifty pounds! He didn't know about his numbers; he just knew that he was here. Not only that he was here, but in his being here in that moment, that time and space, he had one job. And that job was just to breathe. Inhale. Exhale repeat. I believe very much that his parents, and many NICU parents get their strength from doing the same. What can one do at such an unimaginable moment? Control one of the few things that you can at that time. Pause. Be Still. Inhale and then exhale. Just breathe—you and your baby are going to need your oxygen for the moments to come. Maybe even ask the medical time to be quiet for just a second so you can breathe—we don't give parents enough space to do that. I am working hard to do this better.

I think our own lives are very much the same, but sometimes we get sidetracked by the numbers. I wonder what would happen if we chose to keep on moving despite the numbers! Keep on breathing! Keep on kicking and gasp, A NEW SONG! Who knows, we might find out that we like the new song, *and* the new numbers. How cool would that be? Go for it why don't you? If a fourteen-ounce human can do it, so can we!

13

Signs, Symptoms, and Wonders: You Know More Than You Think

"I've learned that I still have a lot to learn."

MAYA ANGELOU

One of the fascinating parts of transition from medical student to intern doctor is the moment that words, symptoms, and diseases on paper begin to represent a true illness in a real live person and not just an answer on a medical school exam or a national board exam for licensing. We spend quite a bit of time learning an incredible amount of information during medical school and residency, and an equally lengthy amount of time regurgitating this information for the stages of medical rounds, grand rounds, and patient case reports. We want to make sure everyone knows that we learned this information. We want to make sure everyone knows that we can adequately explain this information. Most of all, we want to make sure that what we've learned from our patients will empower us to provide even better care for the next patient.

But you don't realize when you're a brand spanking new doctor on the wards at once empowered and petrified that all of the words, lessons, and exams will one day not just be a jumble of flashcards and rainbow highlighters but the best mental rolodex ever in the often-elusive art of medicine. I was halfway through my internship when my rolodex began to form.

In the emergency room while taking a history, I noticed a scarlet sandpaper rash, swollen joints and inquired about history of fever, and realized that group A Streptococcus was real. I also learned that scarlet fever was real, and that pharmacology was actually very important. Well, I already knew it was important but that class had been pretty hard for me. So many medications, and receptors, and side effects, I actually had kind of hoped that I would never have to prescribe a medication ever!

I remembered being in the nursery and being called to examine a newborn who was shaking, according to the nurse. I couldn't believe it. The baby actually had rhythmic, jerking of the left arm. I placed my hand on his arm and it kept moving. I felt the muscle contracting and relaxing beneath my hand. I remember all I had learned about distinguishing seizures from the normal infant startle reflex. I remembered the medications to treat seizures. I watched the face too for simple seizures like lip smacking, eye blinking or tongue fasciculations (when the tongue ripples like a wave), and I remembered the first line treatments like Ativan and phenobarbital. I was pretty proud of myself for remembering, and grateful to help the baby who taught me that seizures were real not just an algorithm in my neurology pathway.

What of my very first premature baby delivery? I mean, my entire life I had prepared for this moment. It was what I knew I was placed on Earth to do. But could I do it? Pediatrics is hard enough. You have to know everything that could happen from newborn to age twenty-one. That's quite a long time period, and a whole lot happens between infancy and adulthood, both normal and abnormal. But neonatal-perinatal medicine adds an additional layer of complexity and asks you to know everything that happens when a human is born too soon, or a human is born amidst challenges and complications, some known but many unknown. That's also a whole bunch of stuff. Yes, stuff, and it's quite daunting.

But when I attended my first delivery for a premature baby, I couldn't believe that I was actually getting to do this. I remember being in the operating room and standing rapt at attention at the warmer. Talking with my right and left hands, the respiratory therapist, and my neonatal resuscitation nurse, I can do nothing without my team, we go through the steps I have reviewed in my head so many times and practiced even more during our Neonatal Resuscitation Program (NRP) certification. Is the temperature okay in the delivery room? Preemies need to be delivered in a warm operating room, which means everyone else might sweat for a minute or two. Is the radiant warmer bed where the baby will be resuscitated on? Is our oxygen ready and working? Is our suction ready and working? Do we have the right breathing tube and the right laryngoscope? Do we have a warm mattress pack and now a saran wrap bag to keep the baby warm? Do we have the appropriate umbilical lines and medications just in case things go differently than planned? Today I can do these steps in my sleep. They are part of my DNA. But that first delivery I was mouthing the steps out loud, making sure our new little friend knew that we were ready, willing, and able to welcome them into our world.

I remember holding my breath for the time out and proudly saying my name as the recording nurse documented my name as part of the medical team. Me, part of the medical team. And then the surgeon made the first abdominal incision or cut. The baby was one and a half pounds, or around 700 grams, and twenty-six weeks, or around six months gestation. A cute little baby girl who came out crying, kicking, and screaming. I looked at her skin as we gently patted her and placed her in her bag for warmth. It was shiny and translucent. I looked at her breast buds, genitalia and at her foot for creases because all of that is part of estimating the maturity of a baby. In this case we had mother's dates from her prenatal care, but many times we do not have that, so we estimate their maturity by doing a Ballard exam and documenting physical and neurologic features. I had done hundreds of them in newborn nursery, but this was my first time doing one on such a tiny baby.

I watched her rib cage go in and out as we placed a nasal CPAP mask over her nose. I couldn't believe that at least for the time being she would not need a breathing tube. I watched her heartbeat beneath the skin of her left chest. I watched her dad's tears trickle down his face as she grabbed one of his fingers with her tiny hands. It was almost as if she said, "It's going to be okay everybody. I'm here. And we can do this." She taught me a lot about being a doctor that day. A big part of my job is to be prepared. But an even bigger part of my job, especially in the world of the NICU and the Land of Labor and Delivery is to wait for the patient to show me the way. They will show me what they need. Sometimes it's emergency intervention. Sometimes it's just time. Sometimes it's to start all over. Sometimes it's to pause and say goodbye. It looks different every time and you have to be a very good dance partner to engage in this dance. No one has time to fight about who is leading or to step on toes. That's okay initially, but if you really want to enjoy the dance you have to figure out really quickly how to stay on beat and enjoy the ride. That's what my patients and families have taught me. Most of all, how to enjoy the ride, and that yes, I can do this. For that I am grateful.

14

Thomas the Train, Dinner, Blue Jeans, and Funerals: When Patients Become Family

"Cure sometimes, treat often, comfort always."

HIPPOCRATES

Over the course of my journey to become a physician, I have attended more lectures than I can count about the intricacies of the patient physician relationship and the imaginary lines that must not ever be crossed. But this is easier said than done. Physicians, nurses, and health care providers often meet patients at their worst, their most vulnerable, in the midst of unbearable brokenness, and they need a healer and a friend. It's hard to do one without the other but even harder when you don't realize which one you are.

A certain objectivity is required to deliver medical news of the facts, the prognosis, the treatment program, and expected trajectory of the case. Of course, we don't have a crystal ball, but patients want to have some idea of what we know so that they can be prepared on some level, which looks different for different families. This transfer of information also requires a certain level of connection with the patient, a knowingness around how your patient likes to receive information. Do they want all the facts? Every detail? Or do they just want the big picture? It's hard to know this without also being a friend, without having spent some time in conversation and reflection to learn what gives a person strength, what gives them joy, and how they navigate life's challenges. We do the same with our friends and family. Some want to know every single thing about our day; others tell us lovingly, but firmly, "just the facts, please, I don't have all day, and it doesn't take all that!"

So how does one avoid blurring the lines when invited into the spaces of intimacy with strangers who become patients during a time when they need a friend and a healer the most? Very delicately and very intentionally. But honestly, I have to admit that I struggle with this more than most. At my core, I am an empath. I'm very touchy-feely. I have a big personality and big energy. I think patients are enveloped by it whether they want to be or not, which I kind of feel bad about! I call it the Dr. Terri experience. It begins with Hi I'm Dr. Terri and I have the pleasure of caring for you child today. Tell me their name. It almost always ends with, "I know we didn't plan for this today, but we are going to get through it together. Congratulations on the birth of your baby." Invariably, after a couple of days, it ends with, "How is it going, Boo?" or "See you tomorrow, Boo," or "Boo, we need to talk." Why? Because I'm from Louisiana and I happen to call everyone, and I mean everyone, Boo. Most people smile. Sometimes they laugh, but after a week of working with me, everyone wanted to be called Boo, and if I didn't call them Boo, they often asked me why they weren't a Boo, too.

It is with that lens I share the first time the lens for me became blurred with respect to patient and provider. Charlotte was a delightful three-year-old little girl with red hair and freckles. She was the first child of one of my favorite sets of parents here referred to as James and Linda. Linda and I hit it off immediately. We were only five years apart in age and I think she looked at me both maternally and sisterly. I was a brand-new intern at age twenty-seven, and she was a new mom at age thirty-two.

Charlotte was a very healthy and playful child with a delightful childhood full of trucks, tumbling, bugs, and Thomas the Train. Her parents affectionately called her Charlie and referred to her as the original tomboy. She became sick one week prior to admission with fever, mild respiratory symptoms, and a rash that was initially felt to be a routine childhood viral infection. Her fevers persisted and she was noted to have a red throat and some joint swelling, with some concern for strep throat and scarlet fever, so she was started on penicillin. Her skin started peeling after seven days, she became more swollen with decreased urine output, inflammation of both of her eyes, and with the brightest red lips like cherries. She was admitted to the hospital due to concerns for possible Kawasaki syndrome.

That is how I met Charlotte, Linda, and James. She was my first introduction to Kawasaki syndrome, an illness common in young children that causes inflammation of the vascular system leading to failure of the heart and kidneys. It is notorious for imitating other illnesses and leading to death due to delayed diagnosis and treatment. Prior to meeting Charlie, the only thing that Kawasaki meant to me was a motorcycle, and now all I think about is Charlotte and her sweet family, and how much I hate the disease. Even years later when the spectrum of a Kawasaki disease-like illness was introduced as part of the array of constellations associated with children infected with COVID, I was reminded of Charlie and her family.

So, I took care of Charlotte, Linda, and James. I learned about Kawasaki disease. I knew every sign and symptom. I reviewed her history over and over, learning how easy it is to confuse it with all the other childhood viral illnesses associated with a rash, and how easy it is to miss. I learned that no matter how many antibiotics you give, sometimes it just doesn't work. I leaned steroids don't fix everything, even if you give higher and higher doses and pray with all of your might, and then some. In the midst of all of that learning, I learned that parents do become friends, and sometimes lines are blurred.

Linda and I would talk every day about how Charlotte was doing and if she was getting better or worse. We would sing her songs and read her stories about her beloved Thomas the Train. We would make choo-choo noises and then laugh at ourselves and discuss the patience of Charlotte. Linda would ask me how internship was going. She would worry about whether I was eating or sleeping enough. She thought this twenty-four-hour call thing was quite ridiculous and couldn't believe it was legal. When I began to lose weight from not eating or sleeping due to the stressors of internship, she lamented about how big my scrubs were and insisted on bringing me a pair of her gently worn jeans. I laughed because I was always complimenting her on her cute jeans and even cuter shape, and we were practically the same size. It's no wonder she felt I needed a pair.

Ten days into her illness, it was apparent that Charlotte was not going to survive. She had drifted into a sleep from which she would not return, almost like Sleeping Beauty, but not quite, because she was not cursed. She was, however, a patient for whom Kawaski this time had won, and we had unfortunately lost. I was not working the next day when Charlotte passed, but her mother sent word to me by one of my friends regarding the funeral arrangements. She had asked that everyone bring something related to

Thomas the train: a book, a toy, or clothing. She planned to donate them all in honor of Charlotte. I thought it was perfectly fitting for such an amazing little girl with even more amazing parents. She was indeed a little engine that could do big things, and I loved the way her parents loved her and the medical team.

We most certainly were not their responsibility, but they welcomed us into their journey of hope and loss, healing, and honor. I learned a lot from Charlotte and her family. Most of all, I learned that sometimes the lines are blurred between patient and physician, and sometimes this blurring is necessary for self-care of the patient and the provider. Thank you to Charlotte, Linda, and James, who taught me about Thomas the Train, jeans, and the parts of the art of medicine that we can't find in the textbooks or classrooms. For that I am grateful.

15

You're Not Okay: When Families See Through Your Superhero Cape

"Grief, I've learned, is really just love. It's all the love you want to give, but cannot. All that unspent love gathers up in the corners of your eyes, the lump in your throat, and in that hollow part of your chest. Grief is just love with no place to go."

JAMIE ANDERSON

If you were to read my personal statement for medical school that was submitted during the fall of 1988 you would find that my primary motivation for wanting to be a physician was to be the kind of doctor that took care of the babies in plastic boxes. The babies that could fit in the palm of your hand like my sister. To have a role in decreasing the disparities that existed for infant mortality in this country. A country where Black women are three to four times more like to experience an adverse pregnancy outcome and two times more likely to experience preterm birth even with a college degree and access to insurance. You'll also find a lofty quote and a summary of my research experiences in college and summer internships at prestigious places like the Centers for Disease Control and Cornell.

What you will not find will be a discussion of my desire to go into medicine because I want to care for babies and children who will not survive. That was not a part of our medical school training then. We only talked about saving lives at every cost. Death? What was that? Failure of a cure? What was that? Because of this void I was woefully unprepared for my first experiences with death during my hematology/oncology rotation.

I was six months into my internship when I did my first rotation through the hematology and oncology wards. Honestly, I had not thought a lot about hematology and oncology beyond my classes in pathophysiology of disease in medical school where we covered all manner of blood-borne disorders and all manner and types of cancers. Way too many to keep in my mind, and at the time I thought only a few applied to children. Boy, was I wrong, and quite naïve! My first few days on the heme/onc floors were not too bad. I met many children with sickle cell disease who had been admitted for pain crisis or pneumonia. Having trained at a medical school with a special mission to serve the underserved, I felt particularly comfortable in this zone. I was encouraged by the fact that I was doing my part to make sure that our patients were receiving adequate pain management, which is often not the case for patients of color. During week two I met several teenagers with a diagnosis of cancer. Several types of cancer, including leukemias, large tumors, and brain tumors. Many of whom had already received not one, but two bone marrow transplants, and had failed to respond to all medical regimens. Several were on experimental treatment protocols in hopes of having just a little more time if not a cure. Many were only five to ten years younger than me, and it was strange to see and experience mortality through their faces and the stories of their families. I was wholly uncomfortable each day with no way to cope. Everyone else on the medical team seemed to think this was okay. This was the job, business as usual. Some of the patients seemed to think the same.

It was in this space I met one of my favorite patients, Benjamin. He was seventeen years old, and his favorite celebrity was the rapper, Tupac. Benjamin was admitted with relapse and diffuse disease after progression of his colorectal cancer. He had failed all therapies and was comfortable with the fact that he was going to die. He wanted to live his life to the fullest until he could no more, and when he could not, he wanted everyone to make sure he was pain free. When we first met, I often talked to both him and his mom. We sang Tupac songs. He shared the latest dances with me and laughed at the fact that I had not heard any of the uncensored Tupac songs. When his care transitioned from curative to comfort, something changed in me. I could no longer go into his room to talk to him or his mother. Deep inside, I felt they had given up. I didn't understand at the time that how he wanted to die was actually something that Benjamin could control.

I begin to present his case outside of the room. I shared numbers and updates. My attending would nod, and we would move on to the next patient. I was ready for that rotation to be over, but I had one more, long week to go. One day after rounds, the hospital chaplain came and found me. He introduced himself and said, "Hi Dr. Major-Kincade, I'm Paul the Chaplain. I wanted you to know that we have a support group for residents that many find helpful. It meets on Tuesdays at 6:30 p.m. Would you like to join?"

I said, "No I don't think so, I'm doing fine. I'm okay."

He said, "Well, Dr. Major-Kincade, Benjamin's mother says you're not. She's worried about you. She says you use to come in and talk to them but that you don't do that anymore. That you stand outside of the room and leave as quickly as you can. That your light is gone."

I was literally shocked. How could she think that I was not okay? I was definitely okay! What did she mean not okay? They were the ones that were not okay after all they had given up not me. And there it was—my inability to handle this situation, the utter futility of medicine, and the betrayal I felt that they had moved on and I had not, I could not. Benjamin's mother was right. I was not okay.

How gracious of her to see that in me during all she was dealing with as a mother. On the verge of losing her son, she wanted to make sure that I was okay. She knew what I had only just learned—that as doctors, we don't wear bulletproof capes, and in the midst of challenges, sometimes our capes do a pretty poor job of protecting us from the fact that we are human. She gave me space to admit that I was not okay, and it has made me a better doctor. For that I am grateful.

16

Is This Really What I Want to Do?
Or Can I Just Drown?

"In this hollow I do grieve for all the things that cease to be."

ANGIE WEILAND-CROSBY

As I've shared through much of this book, I really, really, really wanted to be a doctor—a baby doctor. The kind that took care of the babies in the plastic boxes. The babies that could fit in the palms of your hands. The neonatologists—the preemie baby doctors. I imagined in my mind my own little world of cute little babies in my hands that I would take care of and help to grow and keep safe and comfortable in their plastic boxes until their parents were able to take them home. However, the actual work of medicine, the non-glamorized portion, is this world of those who wear the white coats.

My vision of a world immersed in medicine had no pages that included continuous twelve- and twenty-four-hour work shifts, time away from family, missed meals, or nonexistent bathroom breaks. No vision of families who didn't always appreciate or see your attempts to help them. No vision of co-workers who didn't always see every patient as worthy of the same standard of care. Hospital systems that can offer so little, not designed for those who need so much. There were no pages about the high rates of physician suicide or depression and burn out or compassion fatigue. And there definitely weren't any pages about the amount of debt I would accumulate after having attended college on a full scholarship. These were difficult revelations, and they kept on coming. Sometimes, my friends, your best is actually not good enough! Sometimes, your all falls just a little short because, in fact, we are human, and medicine is not an exact science, despite all of our attempts to convince ourselves otherwise.

I experienced my first bout with depression during the beginning of my third year of medical school. It descended upon me slowly. In between exams, long study halls by myself, and long periods of time away from my family. I was under the impression at the time that depression meant a person who cries all day, but I have come to understand that crying all day is only one form of depression and isn't actually the most common symptom. I had trouble sleeping, trouble eating, and spent long periods in my room sitting in the darkness and stillness in my hammock chair. I wondered, "Is this really what I want to do? Be tired all the time? Be sad all the time? Be dreading work all the time? Be guilty of wanting to sleep? To eat? To pee?" I was only a third-year medical student. If I really planned to be a neonatologist, I still had eight more years to go, and something told me those eight years were only going to get harder!

It was my mother and my best friend, Caroline, from medical school who single-handedly rescued me from this bout of depression. My mother has an uncanny knack to call at just the right time. I am convinced that there is imaginary umbilical cord that has remained in place even after fifty years. She called and said, "Hi Precious! Are you okay?" Of course, I was not, but could only cry as the words would not come. She talked to me only the way a mother could, and I immediately felt loved, safe, not alone, and was reminded that coming to Los Angeles for medical school when my entire support system was in Baton Rouge, Louisiana was probably not my smartest decision or finest moment! The second thing that happened was my best friend from medical school threw me a surprise Pretty Woman birthday party.

She had tried in vain for many days and weeks to get me to leave the apartment, or even my bedroom for that matter, but I would not because the darkness was my friend. Since I could see no light at the end of the tunnel, I was happy to remain where I was. But she did get me to go to the store with her one day because I needed to restock. You can only sit in the darkness eating water and crackers and chocolate for so long, and then you need ice cream. When we returned from the store and went into my apartment, I found all of my friends from medical school were there—and yep, they screamed, "Surprise!" I was amused at how excited their presence made me because in general I truly do hate surprises. They are the ultimate stressor to my constant need for control.

I had seen the movie *Pretty Woman* the year before and was obsessed with the modern-day fairytale. It quickly became one of my favorite movies of all time. My girlfriend Caroline had arranged for the apartment to be decorated with balloons and streamers, she had a basket of all my favorite things, and most importantly, a VHS of the *Pretty Woman* movie and a cassette tape of the soundtrack. I couldn't stop smiling or dancing. And slowly, step by step, with a little help from Julia Roberts, my sweet friend pulled me the rest of the way out of the darkness.

My second experience with depression would come halfway into my internship year. As I shared earlier, I wondered a lot about what my life would be like once I had completed my post-graduate training. Medical school had been pretty intense, and it was just a trial run. Internship and Residency were going to be even more intense and then finally as an Attending, all the gloves were coming off. I didn't have any role models who seemed to be happy with both their professional and personal lives. It seemed everyone was choosing either or and I wanted to be happy doing both. Was that even a possibility? I was staring to believe that perhaps it was not, and that made me very sad.

One day, in the midst of driving to work for my critical care ICU rotation, I started pondering my escape. I was tired of spending the night at the hospital every fourth day for twenty-four hours. I was tired of being sleep deprived. I was tired of running all over the hospital to find patients, clinics, and labs. I was tired of sleeping an hour here or there, stretching my bladder to capacity, and living off peanut butter, graham crackers, and Jell-O cups from the patient snacks. I was tired of presenting numbers, names, histories, plans, and differentials to my attendings when they already knew their plan. I often wondered why they couldn't just tell me the plan, save some time so we could take care of the patient, and maybe one of us could get some sleep—namely me. But I had a lot of guilt about these feelings. After all, I chose this. No one forced me to apply to medical school or to choose this career. And what of the parents and their sick children? They deserved someone fresh and chipper and grateful to be their everyday—grateful to have the opportunity to give it their very best. I wanted to be that person, I just didn't know if I could ever get there, and that worried me a lot!

Not having a break was what bothered me the most. This was before the residency hour rules and time sheets and focus on self-care. This was the time of "I did it so can you. Suck it up buttercup." Certainly, we had vacation up to four weeks per year, but in the interim we could expect to work seven to fourteen days at a time with one or two weekends off each month and a twenty-four-hour call every fourth day. And that, my friends, was going to be your life for at least three years until training was completed. For some reason, on my drives to work, I started thinking what a cool life Rumpelstiltskin must have had because he got to sleep forever. I wanted to sleep forever. It just felt easier than having to walk through the fog of call and chronic fatigue.

One of the things that had weighed heavily on my mind since the start of internship was the story about Susan Smith (History.com, 2021). A mother who, in October of 1994, had killed her two children by allowing her car to roll into a lake with her two children still inside, and then later saying a black man had hijacked her car and kidnapped her kids. As a person of color, I thought a lot about the implications of her lie. I thought a lot about the implications of her crime as a mother and all the others I see daily who can do nothing to save their children who are dying from untreatable diseases. And, I thought a lot about the soothing calmness of water, and later terror as it swallowed up the car and eventually the children. I hoped that they didn't suffer.

On my ride to work every day, I rode across a bridge over a large lake. I often negotiated with myself about the pros and cons of driving into the lake. I was a newlywed and I knew my husband would be devastated. I was the eldest of my parents' three children and from a large family of aunts, uncles, cousins, and grandparents on both sides. I knew that they too would be devastated. But they would find their way. Families have to do this every day, surely mine could too. But sadly, what I was worried about even more than that was the fact that one of my equally tired and possibly depressed co-interns would have to cover my shifts. I couldn't kill myself on a Friday because then someone would have to work and extra weekend— and they needed their weekend off. And I absolutely did not want to be referred to as an annoying afterthought. You know, like, "Dang, why couldn't Terri kill herself on a Monday? Now someone has to work extra this weekend!" Now I really hoped that no one actually would feel that way, but remember, I was in a dark place and not thinking clearly. But I was thinking clear enough to share these thoughts with my husband.

At that time, we only had one car so when our schedules conflicted, he often drove me to work. I actually loved that because I hated driving and still do. In my next life I really need a chauffeur—it's really the only thing on my forever wish list! The hospital where I trained had an amazing entryway with an elaborate train scape. It was like a magical welcome into a world dedicated to children. I used to watch it for hours and would imagine riding the training all over the city. Walking past it always made me smile. But lately, just entering the building brought tears to my eyes. The effort to lift my feet up and down and move myself forward actually felt like walking through a fog of molasses and quicksand, and it seemed to be getting harder and harder. My sweet husband knew that I was tired, but he had no idea that I was becoming increasingly depressed and pondering suicide. He hugged me and looked into my eyes and said the sweetest words I have ever heard. "Baby I love you. If you don't want to be a doctor anymore that's fine. You can do something else. It's not worth it. It's okay to change your mind." Now he said exactly what I needed to hear, and at that moment, I knew that I did still want to be a doctor, but I was not okay. Also, I knew I kind of still needed to be a doctor! I personally had over two hundred thousand dollars in debt from my medical school education!

We made an appointment with my department chair to address my mental health concerns. He was an amazing man and I felt like I knew him well. He had handpicked each one of us for our residency class. He met with us immediately, listened to us, validated us, and told us that not only that we were going to be okay, but that we were not alone. He referred me to a therapist who worked with residents who had depression. She helped me with processing, coping, and my depression, and briefly treated me with meds. I was grateful. That was twenty-one years ago, and I have never looked back. His willingness to validate me and our willingness to acknowledge that we were not okay did wonders for my approach to my self-care as a physician. More importantly, I have become the physician I aspired to be—happy to go to work every day, happy for the privilege to meet and share with families, happy to work with likeminded colleagues who inspire me, and happy at work and at home. For me, it doesn't get much better than that, so I will continue to savor every moment because it's okay to not be okay!

17

Hypocrisy of the NICU: Rules and Regulations for Parent Visitation

"Until you have a preemie you never understand the great distance between one pane of glass."

PREMATURE BABIES AND BEYOND FACEBOOK GROUP

When you have a baby that is admitted to the Neonatal Intensive Care Unit you get an immediate stamp on your passport to a place where parents are parents, but not really. When you imagine being a parent, it means at a minimum you expect to have control over basic things like when you can pick up your child and put them down, what you feed your child and how you feed them, and who can visit your child and who cannot visit your child. These are choices we take for granted in the world of parenthood. On a bigger level, we expect to control what treatments or procedures our child can or cannot have, how long we would expose them to certain treatments, when they need to see a doctor, and when they do not. After all, their well-being is our priority, and parents are in the best position to determine their future well-being.

However, in the NICU, all of those inherent roles are immediately thrown into question, and parents have to learn to navigate and rally one-by-one to be advocates for their children and true partners in their care.

For most babies in the Neonatal Intensive Care Unit (NICU), we determine their arrival from the time of delivery. Sure, some come to us later from the newborn nursery after having initially being stable and later becoming unstable, or even going home with a missed infection or major defect like a heart problem, or even jaundice which often shows up late. For those we may meet them in the nursery several days later during their first week of life, but for most of our precious cargo, usually related to a breathing problem that does not get better or a birth defect that will require subspecialty care, we determine their destiny at delivery.

This decision to take a baby to the Neonatal Intensive Care Unit (NICU) is the decision that disrupts the parent-child relationship. Embedded in our delivery of this announcement is the imperative that we are now in charge because your baby needs us. Your baby needs us more than your baby needs you at this time, and that's a pretty hard pill to swallow when you have waited what seems like a lifetime to meet this new cherished family member. We stabilize your baby at delivery, and if we're lucky, you're lucky, and the baby's lucky, we get a moment to bring your baby to your face so that you can say hello. Smell their hair, nuzzle their nose, count their fingers and toes. Sometimes, we also get to grab a quick family picture. It may be the only picture that some families receive. Then we say, "Okay we need to take your baby to the NICU now. We need to run some tests, check some numbers. We will find you later to give you an update. Congratulations!" Then we disappear with your baby.

Notice that we are not asking you if your baby can come with us, we are telling you that your baby is coming with us, and if they are able to, we invite your partner to follow us along the way to the NICU to capture the moment for you. I have said this statement to so many families, so many times. It never gets easier, but I have to say it anyway because my job is to take care of your baby, and I hope with all my heart that I'll be able to make up for the moments you lost in the delivery room with moments of life in the NICU. But I never know how it is going to work out.

I often wonder what parents think about at that moment. I mean, beyond hoping and praying that their child is going to be okay, because everyone wants that. But what do they think about the transfer of power of roles in the care of their child, or do they even have time to think about it all? I know from the literature that most do not because they are in a period of profound shock, but I still wonder how we could do any of this better.

This change in direction of roles with parents becoming less primary and the medical team becoming more primary continues with our welcome to the NICU speech. "Hi, this is the NICU. Take off your watch, Fitbit, and jewelry. Place it and your cell phone in these zip lock bags because you have germs that could make your baby sick. Your things have germs that could make your baby sick. Now wash your hand for twenty seconds. You know, sing the Happy Birthday Song twice, don't forget the elbows and between the fingers and underneath the fingernails. I have to keep your baby safe. Safe from you. Now can you sign these forms, forms that cover a bunch of procedures that you may not even remember us talking about the next day, but you sign them anyway because you want the best for your baby, and we have told you that we are the best for your baby."

"Now it's time to verify that the ID bands you received at delivery are on your wrist. Keep them on forever. Never ever, ever, take them off because this is how you will get to see your baby. This is how we verify that you are actually the parent for this baby. Who would you like to be able to visit? Write their names here. Then we show you where your baby is in the NICU. They may be on a radiant warmer bed with the top up so you can see them and touch them or they may be inside of an incubator or isolette, where you can open little portholes to see them and touch them. But not of course till we the NICU medical team tell you that you can touch them."

Now comes my biggest pet peeve about the NICU rules and regulations—the touch times. Premature babies and sick term babies are very fragile, very sensitive to touch. This means sometimes when we touch them, they can drop their heartrates very low and their oxygen even lower. Sometimes they even stop breathing. It's risky business touching these babies, but we have to as a part of their care. But somewhere along the line, we decided our touch was a necessary inconvenience for their care and healing in a way the touch of parents is not. That really bothers me. And it still bothers me. I have talked to so many parents over the years who just wanted to see their baby, touch their baby, even hold their babies, but were told that their baby was too unstable to do that for this visit. Maybe try again in the next shift, the shift twelve hours away.

Don't get me wrong, I really do think that most parents, if not all parents, can understand that if they have a very sick baby, they may not be able to hold them. In fact, many of them would rather die than to do anything that would cause their child to be more unstable, and sometimes we have to beg them to even touch the baby because they are so afraid. But to not be able to touch a finger, stroke a lock of hair, or scrape the bottom of one tiny foot with just the gentlest touch of a fingernail when the medical team is doing heel sticks with needles for blood draws, tourniquets on the arms for intravenous lines or needles though the chest for emergency lung collapse, it just doesn't make sense. And I am unable to reconcile the difference between the two and the necessary imposition of one intervention over the other.

What about for infants who are no longer critically ill but just in the illustrious category of feeding and growing? The babies who parents can hold or do kangaroo care with. That cherished time of skin to skin or being held chest to chest often when they are receiving food through their feeding tubes. Most premature or sick babies eat every three hours. Parents get used to those schedules. They arrange their lives by those schedules. It's a time to not only feed the baby, but often parents are able to change the diapers then and take their baby's temperature. They get to do parent things. So, imagine being a working mom whose baby has already been in the ICU nursery for two months who finally has a baby stable enough to hold every day. Imagine having to go back to work before your baby is discharged home but arranging your schedule so you can hold your baby every day for the 6:00 a.m. feeding and touch time before you go to work, and the joy you feel at having that little corner of parenthood, motherhood, or fatherhood on lock. Then imagine coming into the NICU and being told by a new staff member that your baby has already been fed because they have too many babies and since your baby doesn't really take a bottle it was easiest to do the feed early. Of course, they apologize because they didn't know you come every morning at 6:00 a.m. even though you've come every morning at 6:00 a.m. for the past four weeks and there are signs around the room that say please wait for my mommy, daddy, or designated loved one to feed me.

These are the situations that drive me crazy. When I'm called to the bedside not to discuss a child that's critically ill, but rather a parent of a child who is stable who has been told, or in this case shown, once again that they aren't the parent. That they are not in control. That they can't even control the most basic of things like if they can expect consistency for when they come to visit their baby who is now stable. After twenty-plus years in the world of neonatal care, I am clear that sometimes things just don't work out. We make all the best plans, and the babies decide they have other plans, so we just try to keep up. Sometimes, we don't have enough nurses or doctors, but we try our best. The babies don't care. They are there and they demand our best even when our best is stretched pretty thin. That's our problem, not theirs. But when things do get out of control, we owe it to our families to be proactive when telling them why things are changed. Why we couldn't honor their wishes that day and how we will work to honor them the next time. At the very least, we need to make sure parents know and understand that their child is a valued patient of ours, one for whom we have individualized care. Their child is not just a patient in a NICU who is a line item in a policy, all black and white without grays and definitely no colors. Most of all, we want to remember that they are the parent, we are not, and they are valued members of our medical team.

Let's not change plans without making sure every member of the medical team is aware. It may not seem like a big deal, but for me, I will never forget the mom who left the NICU crying on her way to work because someone decided that her touch time, her kangaroo time before work during her child's team feeding, was not worth accommodating one Friday morning. At the end of the day, we all just want to know we matter. That goes for the babies and the children, and I thank every NICU parent for teaching me that. Now that I too am a parent of a child with special needs, I understand even more the importance of embodying every aspect of my role as a parent. I also want that for my NICU parents, and it starts with the delivery room, where the children remind you that you may be the medical team, but you are not their parent. How easily we forget!

18

Saying Hello and Goodbye: Finding a Moment to Just be a Mom

"You were unsure which pain is worse—the shock of what happened or the ache for what never will."

SIMON VON BOOY

In the past 20 years I've met many angels in the NICU—some in the form of one-pound babies, most in the form of the humans they call mom or dad. The hardest part of my job by far is taking a moment to talk to a family about the things we really don't want to talk about—the things no parent should have to talk about: that despite all of our efforts their child may not survive. Or sometimes because of our efforts their child will survive but will be significantly devastated physically and neurologically. There's no easy way to have those conversations but what I know for sure is that every family deserves our honest opinion. It's the very least we can do as they process what choice is best for their family, and many times the choice is really no choice at all. How do you choose between doing everything and almost everything when the results of those choices may leave your child here physically but absent socially, developmentally, and mentally? I want to scream when we as providers pretend that these are choices. But after I'm done screaming, I move forwards slowly, quietly, and intentionally to meet our families where they are, and I wait patiently for them to teach me more about this thing we call life; this journey we call parenthood; and this experience of physical love, pain, and sacrifice. They teach me something every single day.

I am particularly reminded of lessons learned from a very special family that I'd like to share here. The first is the story of a beautiful baby girl born three weeks early; her name was Anna. She was the second child for her parents but the first premature baby. By our accounts, this two-and-a-half-pound baby girl was a giant in the world of premature infants. As with many preemies, she announced her arrival into the world very suddenly. Her mom, Susan, had seen her OB early that morning, and everything was fine. They had taken 3D ultrasound pictures and were already in love with Anna's fat cheeks and crinkly nose. It appeared as if Anna was already in love with her fingers, especially her thumb, which she was always sucking. I'm always amazed when I see the babies sucking their thumbs on the ultrasound. It's a pretty direct reminder that human development is pretty awesome and always evolving. So many of things we associate with occurring only after delivery are just continuation of things that were occurring in utero.

Shortly after leaving her morning appointment with her obstetrician, Susan returned home to finish an exciting day of nesting and getting things ready for her baby. While at home, her water broke and she called her husband, Adam, who was equally and understandably overwhelmed with this news. After all, their baby wasn't due for another three months. They were only twenty-eight weeks pregnant. Susan delivered shortly after arriving at the hospital, and Anna was rushed immediately to the NICU. Unfortunately, we did not get to meet Susan or Adam prior to the delivery. Not that we always have a chance to meet new NICU moms and dads, but we try very hard to—just to have a conversation about what's to come, what to expect, and to validate that what is happening is real, because for so many it never feels real. No one signs up for the roller coaster ride that is the NICU but once you find yourself there, you just have to buckle the seatbelt and hold on, whether you're tall enough for the ride or not. It's quite frightening even for those of us who have chosen it as our life's profession, and it never gets easier.

Unfortunately, despite being a very good size preemie, Anna was very sick and didn't respond to any of our fancy breathing machines or strong heart and lung medications or fancy antibiotics. Yes, we were able to keep her heart beating for several days, but her body was getting tired. We saw less of her each day and more wires. What's worse is that because she came so fast and was so sick at delivery, her parents had never gotten to hold her. One of my biggest pet peeves is when teams don't take the time to make sure the parents get to see the baby before we leave the delivery room, to kiss the top of their forehead, to count fingers and toes, and to grab a quick family picture, because sadly it may be the only picture many of them ever receive. In Anna's case, Susan and Adam had only been able to see their baby very briefly because she was so sick and needed to get to the NICU to stabilize her heart rate and oxygen.

By day three of her short and courageous life, it was clear that Anna was not going to survive. Her heart rate was getting slower and slower, her oxygen was getting lower and lower, and her blood pressure becoming fainter and fainter. Susan and Adam had asked us to continue to fight for Anna until the very end, which we were committed to doing, but it was getting harder and harder. We have so many wonderful machines and medicines in the NICU but for each intervention there is a tradeoff. Sometimes they work without any problems. I love it when that happens. Other times, they work but leave immediate consequences, and sometimes they leave long-lasting consequences when they don't recover for years if at all—all in the name of saving a life. It's a very difficult place to navigate, as we're saving babies we wouldn't have been able to save twenty, fifteen, or even as recently as ten years ago. I'm so grateful that most of the babies we care for will turn out fine, but I'm daily reminded of the sacrifices made by the babies and the families who don't have those stories of survival to share. Rather, they have a different type of story, a story that begins with hello and ends with goodbye.

On the day Anna died, we tried CPR three times before she and her parents both decided enough was enough. There were lots of tears by the parents as well as the staff. We all wanted so badly for Anna to beat the odds, to come back to the NICU reunion when she was one or two years old and remind all of us that every procedure, every day, every alarm, every up and down had been so very worth it. But Anna's story was going to be a different one. I often marvel at these tiny warriors who defy medical odds and hang on for just a couple of days so that their parents get to be parents. Hold their fingers, count their toes, slip a wedding band along their tiny arms, stroke their hair, and kiss their foreheads. It's a beautiful gift and reminds me that there is a greater power and why I love my job so much. I am convinced I am in the presence of angels every day. Some stay with us, some leave us, and other guide us just for the moment. Ask anyone who works in the NICU they will tell you the same!

Often once a child has passed the family needs a moment of privacy alone and then requests uninterrupted time to spend with their child. It's a sacred time, and for many parents it may be the first time either Mom or Dad got to even hold their child. There may be whispered dreams, affirmations of love, expressions of regret all held in a circle of sacred silence. On this day Anna had died late in the afternoon, right before change of shift. We invited the family into our butterfly room and shared that we would bring Anna to them once we had chance to clean her up and remove all of her intravenous lines and wires. I returned to the bedside and watched as our neonatal bereavement team began to remove Anna's wires and leads. She looked so peaceful. I was strangely encouraged that she didn't have bruising all over her chest, which sadly is not uncommon after baby CPR. Once all of her leads were removed, they were just getting ready to bathe her and put her in one of the handmade gowns volunteers made for babies who have passed—in some strange way it gave us all a sense of peace to pick out this last outfit for our special patient.

However, just before that moment, I felt a tap on my shoulder and it was Susan, Anna's mother. She said some words that I will never forget: "Can I bathe her? I never got to hold her. Bathing her will be one way I can feel like her mother. I know you want to clean her up for us, but I would like to do that. Would that be, okay?" I paused.

Everyone paused. Of course, she could bathe her daughter—it's like we all said it at once! In my mind we were cleaning her up to present her, but in this mother's mind we were taking away a rite of passage between mother and daughter at end of life. It was such a simple request, but it spoke volumes and it changed the way we approached end of life care for all our babies and families. We stepped back and left Susan with Anna. She smiled as she approached her daughter. She gently used the baby washcloth to wipe Anna from head to toe and followed that with gently lotioning her before she put on the tiniest preemie diaper and a lovely pale blue christening gown.

We could all hear, see, and feel her joy and I'll never forget the privilege of being witness to such a special and sacred moment. That's the story of hello and goodbye. Each family's story is unique, and I have learned lessons from all of them. I try to make sure that the chapters I write include the especially important lessons I've learned from families like Susan, Adam, and Anna.

19

Why I Believe in Hope

"Remember, hope is a good thing, maybe the best of things, and no good thing ever dies."

STEPHEN KING

Although I don't know what it's like to have a child that was premature or what it's like to experience pregnancy or infant loss, I do know what it's like to have hope despite what man is telling you. I do know what it's like to be in front of a medical or educational professional and be told things about your child's future potential that would give any parent great pause. My own journey with a child with special needs informs me whenever I'm sharing with a family in the NICU who might be facing a future with a child who may have developmental challenges. Yes, it's my job to provide information, but it's not my job to take away hope. In fact, I know without a doubt that in many cases hope is the one thing that allows a family to persevere in spite of their situation, while at the same time allows us, the health care providers, to be inspired by what we do. None of it matters if our babies and families don't leave believing the experience was worth it and that their best is yet to come.

My first pregnancy was relatively uneventful—other than being three years earlier than we planned—but she came on God's timetable, not ours. I was a first year Neonatology fellow and had just finished my three-year Pediatric internship and residency. The fellowship was an intense training period requiring twenty-four-hour call every fourth night for the year and thirty days of clinical service every other month. I would not advise anyone to enter the realm of childbearing during this period. But, as they say, God has a sense of humor! Our baby girl was one month earlier or so I thought (apparently my prenatal care was less than optimal) and was healthy, happy and full of grace. Thank goodness she accepted that her dad and I were the definition of on-the-job training and loved us through it anyway! She's almost twenty-four years old today and halfway through her third year of veterinarian school. We are quite proud of her.

Our son would be born almost three years later, and we planned for him. We were elated to be rounding out our family of four with one boy and one girl—so elated that we even named our children after ourselves! Our son was a sweet, inquisitive baby. He liked things on his time, like his toys organized a certain way, and spent long hours building and drawing. He didn't talk a lot during his early years and when he did, we didn't always understand all of the words he used.

Our son was four years old when we realized that he was different. He was largely non-verbal and enjoyed his company over the company of others. He could play for hours and hours alone and build the most magnificent creations and draw the most imaginative mythical creatures. He wrote all of his letters backward including the letters in his name. We were told initially that his challenges were because he was a late July birthday and that he simply needed to repeat kindergarten but that would not be the case.

These problems magnified in the second year of kindergarten, and he began to also have challenges with numbers and simple math. When we started sight words, he wrote most of them phonetically. We had him formally tested at age six and were told that his primary diagnosis was a speech language processing disorder compounded with a reading disorder. He would later pick up additional labels like sensory integration disorder, dyslexia, dyscalculia, slow processing speed and short-term memory deficits, and he was an auditory learner, which is really hard in a visual classroom filled with lectures and power points. On top of it all we would learn that his IQ was totally normal, so he was not developmentally delayed but he did have several learning disabilities. What did it all mean? I liken it to being a square peg in a round world.

We sought out many resources and were fortunate to live in Dallas, which boasted a claim of being home to several schools for children who learned differently, including a premier school that was nationally ranked. After our formal testing, we sought additional help for our son at several of these schools and were in for a rude awakening. It was hard being a pediatrician and neonatologists, with access to resources, and to hear from multiple resources that my son, our son, was unteachable. One administrator literally looked me dead in the eyes and said, "We have reviewed your son's assessments. Our school cannot help him. We can help kids with one learning issue not multiple. Your son is unteachable and will always struggle." I mean, who says that to a parent? It sent me to a very dark place because I internalized the words of this professional. Thank goodness my husband did not.

We cried. We prayed. We researched. We continue to nurture, encourage and challenge our amazing little boy and eventually we found a place that was a perfect fit for him and his amazing abilities. That was fifteen years ago. Our son went on to do well in a school for children with primary speech and language difficulties. He did well there and was able to transition back to traditional school during middle school. We learned the value of having a 504b accommodation plan and an individualized education plan (IEP), which explicitly listed his accommodations and the best way to ensure success with his style of learning. We attended our admission, review and dismissal (ARD) meeting for his educational goals. We met some amazing teachers who championed for him. He went on to receive a peer advocacy award and several local art awards, be coach of the wrestling team, and receive an honorary induction into the National Honor Society.

Today, our son is a junior in art school pursuing his dream of a career in media and animation. He hopes to one day add Pixar Animator to his roster. Of course, I'm biased, but I believe with all of my heart that anyone would be lucky to have him. He still takes longer to carry out creative tasks than most of his peers, but he does complete them. His confidence is through the roof, and he is quite comfortable with who he is today. As a parent, I have to say that's no small feat given the challenges that he has experienced.

So, when I'm in front of a parent whose child may be facing physical, mental, or developmental issues, I remember the moment that an educator said to me that my child was unteachable. I remember what it felt like to have my hope crushed and dismissed. I remember the missed opportunity to partner alongside me for the moments yet to be seen. The moments that surprise you. The moments that may not meet all of your expectations but that are so much better than the what ifs someone has painted for you.

I don't know all the answers, but I do know it's possible to have hope and to wish for a different outcome at the same time. It's possible to hear the hard truths and still embrace hope. Sometimes it's the only thing we can embrace. We embrace it in our words. In our hearts. In our tears. It's in the nods, the exhales, and the sighs, and the way our very heart beats as we wait for the heartbeats of another to meet us where we are. I hope I never forget that as I'm talking to parents, and I hope they trust me enough to be in the space of hope with them even during hard truths. Because it's on the other side of hope we finally exhale. And that, my friends, is why I love my job. Who wouldn't? Breath of Life, after twenty years of hope, love, and loss, it all comes down to the most obvious remainder of our humanity.

Breathe easy my friends! I look forward to the next twenty years. I hope to see you there.

20

Offering Hope and Bearing Witness: A Mid-Career Change to Pediatric Hospice and Palliative Medicine

"Be a light of hope in the landscapes of a soul."

ANGELICA HOPES

Twenty years into my career and neonatal and perinatal medicine, I decided to pivot and pursue additional training in the field of pediatric palliative care and hospice medicine. I completed the manuscript for this book just before starting this journey. Along the way, many friends and colleagues asked me repeatedly what the heck was wrong with me. The decision to go back to residency in my early fifties, I believe, is the natural culmination of my journey of caring for babies and families. Yet, to many on the outside looking in, I seemed to be on the brink of a psychotic break, and they desperately wanted me to have a mental evaluation and some of the good, good meds.

Honestly, I couldn't blame my friends and family. After all, I finished my neonatology training exactly twenty-one years ago to the date that I was now starting additional training, but this time in Pediatric Hospice and Palliative Medicine. I had been an attending neonatologist for twenty-one years! I had been my own boss. I was in control of my schedule and my destiny. I had built up an array of skills in my filed that afforded me well in caring for babies, interacting with colleagues, and talking to families. And I loved every minute of my job taking care of babies in the plastic boxes as much today as I did twenty-one years ago.

So how did I come to decide that taking care of premature and sick term babies in the NICU was just a prelude to the next step? I don't really feel like I chose pediatric hospice and palliative medicine. I believe with all of my heart that the field chose me. Early in my career I found that I had an ease with talking to families about difficult choices, an ease that many of my colleagues did not have. It seemed like no matter where I worked, babies who had been previously stable would suddenly become unstable and parents would appear and ask hard questions—questions they wanted to ask before but had not been presented the opportunity to discuss. It was a familiar scenario and rationalized by my colleagues, "well, they didn't ask, and we didn't offer." This was particularly concerning in babies who had been critically ill and declining for hours and sometimes days. It was not an infrequent scenario that I would come in for my night shift and be told, "Oh Terri, we are so glad you're here. Can you talk to these parents? They are asking some hard questions," or worse, "Terri, these parents are in denial, can you help get them on the same page?" My immediate reaction would be, "which page is that? Why aren't we on the parent's page? What is their page? Are we even in the same chapter of the same book?" I was amazed at how so much medical mistrust happens as a result of communication failures.

I really don't think there was anything particularly special about the way I approached families, but I do think there was something unique in the way I intentionally held space for them without an agenda. I wanted parents to know that I am here to hear your story, your child's story. I want to know what you understand about your child and what your goals for his or her life may be. I want to know what life you've imagined for your child in light of this current illness and how we can best support that. So much of that involves listening, naming, and honoring.

I called children by their names, not their disease processes. I honored the life that was in front of me and celebrated their presence, sometimes for only minutes or hours, other times for days or weeks. Many times, parents said to me that I was the only one who said their child's name. I was the only one who offered them a path to home because their true wish was to at least be able to take their child home, often to die in their own bed. I was the only one who didn't think it was strange to still want to offer a parent the opportunity to breast feed a child for comfort, even with major birth defects or a chance to place a feeding tube in the nose for a child with major chromosome problems. I hoped with the parents that their baby would defy the odds and actually survive the delivery and dare to leave the delivery room, even when the numbers said they most likely would not. My role was and is to bear witness, nevertheless.

I have saved several cards from early in my career and one of my favorites was a note from a mom whose child was born very premature and only lived three hours, forty minutes, and five seconds. In the card she said, "Thank you for calling Violet by name. Thank you for making sure I got to hold. Thank you for making sure she had the best three hours, forty minutes, and five seconds she could ever have. Because of you her goodbye, though bittersweet, gave us the joy of her complete existence, and we will never forget that." I didn't think about it at the time. In fact, I was so sad that Violet passed so quickly, but that family taught me how important it is to pause and bear witness.

I received a similar note from another family who had been given a very grim prognosis about their extremely premature child and told in no uncertain terms that they needed to stop. They had heard all of the numbers. They understood the prognosis, but they weren't ready to stop, and everyone had made them feel that that was not okay. Again, I happened to be on that night and the charge nurse asked me to talk to the family. I don't even remember what I said, but I did want them to know that if they weren't ready to stop, that was okay. I wanted them to know that they were not bad parents. I wanted them to know that although we the medical team often insist on the urgency of these decisions, many times these decisions are not as urgent as we think, and often the babies will declare themselves.

That baby survived and thrived, and on his one-year birthday, his parents shared that they were in the midst of despair, when the lady with big smile and small afro came to talk to them. They felt that even though I acknowledged how sick their child was, and the rocky road ahead, that somehow, I had managed to leave them with a bit of light, but most of all they were empowered to advocate for their child and the life he would have. It made me smile because I often say I specialize in the gift of hope, but the gift of hope looks different for different families. It's not always rainbows and bunnies, but there is a way to share honest information to empower informed decision making, and the hope and dream that the parents still hold in their hearts. You can plan and hope at the same time. We do at all the time, but for some reason, it makes us a little uncomfortable when parents of critically ill children want to do this.

Over the course of my career, my heart was drawn more and more to families who might have to say hello and goodbye, and my colleagues called me more and more. I remember the families of babies gone too soon, often more vividly than the hundreds of babies that I have sent home who did not die. I started to realize that we will not be able to save every baby (it took me a while to realize this), but we can most certainly endeavor to save the human spirit. And if we can do that, saving the human spirit that is the very best that we can do. Families are going to remember those last moments and those first moments. It's an awful feeling to have been part of process that makes those last moments even worse. I've certainly made my share of mistakes when helping families at the end of life, but I've worked hard to be better. Our families really deserve that. At the moment we know that our patient is not going to survive, it's important to focus on our ability to minimize their suffering, to give them peace as much as we can. There is a saying in palliative care which sounds foreign to those not in the field, but there is no excuse for a bad death. Everyone deserves a good death.

I began to intentionally develop my skills in this area, completing a yearlong training program at Harvard dedicated to palliative care education and practice. This allowed me to return to my practice and help to build our neonatal palliative care teams—meeting families prior to delivery who were carrying babies who might not survive, helping them to carve out their delivery and birth experience, naming how they might have to say goodbye in the event that our biggest fears for realized, talking to families with clear care plans and clear views about quality of life, and helping to navigate choices with the medical team. Naming moral distress and compassion fatigue among colleagues and offering safe spaces to discuss difficult deaths were and are some of the most fulfilling moments of my career. To enter into the sacred space between life and death and sit with the family as they honor and cherish their family members on this side of Heaven while still on Earth is such a gift, and what I've learned from these families is that time matters, words matter, and silence matters.

The field of pediatric palliative care and hospice medicine didn't actually exist as a specialty until 2008. I was already eight years into my perinatal-neonatal medicine career at the time. I already knew I had a passion for patients and families navigating chronic illness, especially at the end of life, but the field didn't exist in 2000, so I had navigated my own way. Once the field became a subspecialty, I debated taking the exam like many of my colleagues, that would allow me to sit for the exam and be a board-certified physician in hospice and palliative Medicine. To be grandfathered in, I would have to spend several months seeing adult hospice patients to have enough deaths to quality for the exam, which I could have done, but I didn't want to do that. I knew that my comfort was babies and parents. But if I really wanted to do this well, I would need formal training and experience with talking to big kids and their parents. Patients who could actually talk back to me. I was both excited and petrified.

I promised myself that I would eventually go back and do the fellowship, but then life happened, and years passed. My kids got older, I got older, and before knew it I was already fifty. Could I really go back to training now? I wasn't sure that I could! I decided to do another educational program, this time in pediatric bioethics, at Mercy Children's Hospital in Kansas City. It was one of the top five educational experiences of my life, and I've had a lot of educational experiences! To devote an entire year to the science of ethics, choices, decision making as it applies to children and parents was fascinating to me, and I learned so much. My world is the world of neonatology, but there were a whole lot of ethical issues beyond neonatology. I was clear at the end of that year that I needed to do the fellowship.

The day before I decided to apply to return to medical training, I receive an early morning phone call at 7:00 a.m. It was Cindy, the mom of a baby who I had only met twice before. Once shortly after delivery and once shortly before discharge home on hospice. She was the mother of beautiful, sweet baby girl named Esther. Esther had freckles and curly reddish blonde hair. Her daughter had been delivered unexpectedly at home and there were complications associated with the delivery. The baby was perfect on the outside in every way—fat cheeks, ten fingers and toes, long eyelashes, the cutest nose. She was a very wanted child but had severe brain injury, and we believed would likely never walk or talk eat or have capacity for joy. But she did breathe. The team had completed a few conversations related to options for care, and I was invited to help them to process their decision making. Many of the options they had previously been presented were final and absolute, like surgeries for tracheostomy and surgery for a gastrostomy tube. They had been offered these options in a way that was non-negotiable, but the family wasn't sure they wanted that. We talked about a bridge to going home like with a feeding tube in the nose, oxygen, and a suction machine, which they greatly appreciated. Having bridges is important for families to navigate their choices, and so often we don't offer bridges, just hard detours.

Cindy wanted me to know that her daughter Esther had passed that morning. But what she mostly wanted to do was to thank me for giving them a bridge to go home. To thank me for connecting them with an outpatient palliative care team. To thank me for introducing the concept of hospice, which they weren't ready for at the time, but when the time came, they were able to make the best decisions for their family because of our earlier conversations. Because of the commitment to holding space and honoring the life of Esther. For me it was a crystal-clear confirmation that I was on the right path. So, I applied for my palliative and hospice medicine fellowship that day and my husband, kids, friends, and family came along for the ride. I can't wait to share what I have learned over the next twelve months. In the meantime, keep holding space. Keep bearing witness. Keep listening. You can thank me later.

Afterword
Full Circle Moments

*"I do not understand the mystery of grace –
only that it meets us where we are and does not leave us where
it found us."*

ANNE LAMOTT

I am not sure if anyone will even read my book, but I had to write it for myself and for the patients and families whom I've been blessed to care for over the first twenty years of my career. It seemed like a particularly pivotal moment given my decision to change careers after twenty years from neonatal and perinatal medicine to pediatric hospice and palliative medicine at the ripe old age of fifty-three.

I'm having a bit of an identity crisis in the midst of this transition. I mean I've been Dr. Terri MD and Dr. Boo the Preemie Doc for the majority of my professional life and most of my adult life, and I'm still trying to figure out who Terri the Pediatric and Hospice Medicine Fellow is. I hope she turns out to be as cool as this version of me because I kind of like her.

I wanted to take a moment to thank those who have been part of the journey. Those who have made me who I am. Those who have taken a moment to allow me a glimpse into their lives as a parent of a sick baby in the neonatal intensive care unit or the parent of a baby gone too soon. Those who have taken the time to come back and say to me, "I appreciated when you did this," or "I didn't appreciate it when you did that." It's made me not just a better doctor but a better human.

I've been practicing medicine long enough now that my former patients are now graduating from high school and going to college. I love getting their graduation cards. It reminds me that our work is not in vain and that miracles are real. They walk, they breathe, they go to high school, and they go on to college. They even message me on Instagram and tell me they were one of my preemie babies and that they plan to pursue a career in neonatal nursing.

I've said it before, but I really do have the best job in the world. My favorite part of my job is going to deliveries and then sending babies home. I am sure I am as happy as they are, if not happier. They deserve to finally get to go home after everything they have gone through, and it means so much to me when they finally are able to do so. It's so much more than a full-circle moment. So hard to describe, but I see the montage of their NICU journeys every time they walk out of the NICU and into the rest of their lives.

Thank you for bringing your children back to our NICU reunion parties. It matters that we see them laughing in your arms. It matters that we see your faces free of worry. It matters that they look at us and smile instead of cry, but who can blame them if they cry, because there are memories that they can never convey from the recesses of their minds. Thank you for the gifts that you bring back to the NICU for other parents and babies—the shirts, the Christmas ornaments, the blankets. Thank you for the snacks for the staff and the reminders that you see us. Thank you for acknowledging that the work we do matters—sometimes it's hard to recognize, especially for those of you who have had to say goodbye to your babies in the NICU. You will always be a part of our families and we will never forget your sweet babies!

To the NICU nurses that have become my NICU besties over the past twenty years—what can I say? Because of you I am! From the very beginning you've held my hand, made sure I had something to eat in the midst of long shifts, and made sure I got a fifteen-minute nap here or there and insisted that no one call me or disturb me unless it was an emergency! You understood my dyslexia and dyscalculia, and always helped me to double-check my orders. You dealt with my attention deficit disorder (ADD) and knew that I had to round alphabetically and in order, and got used to me saying, "I am on the D's. I haven't got to the H patients yet. Please only call for an emergency." Then you made sure other nurses knew that as well.

You brought gifts for my daughter when she was born and hosted a baby shower. You even kept her a couple of times when my husband and I both worked nights. Then, when my son came along, you kept him too. You let me cry on your shoulders when we had a tough delivery and a tough day in the NICU, and we learned and grew together. You really are some of my absolute favorite people and I so appreciate you.

Now to the little humans in the plastic boxes. What can I say that hasn't been said? Thank you for the pleasure of meeting you, for the pleasure of caring for you, for your patience with all the procedures and all of the ups and downs, for your courage and your spunk in defying the odds, for crying in the delivery room when we really needed you to break the silence, for reaching your hand up to your mom and dad when your heard their voice, for growing and getting strong enough to get out of the incubator and into the crib, for spending just a little time with us when you were just passing through and reminding us all that life is precious—measured in moments, experienced in real time. Your mom and dad are the most important people in the world, and hello is just as important as goodbye.

Ode to Preemies from Doctor Boo

Little miracles wrapped in skin

No one understands the power within

We measure your life in weeks and days

But we later experience it in so many ways

Tiny little fighter

Working so hard to breathe

The things you have gone through would bring adults to their knees

You sleep so much your parents wonder if something is wrong

But we know that sleeping allows you to heal and hopefully grow strong

So many ups and downs on this roller coaster ride

But eventually you hit your stride

I think I hold my breath as much as you

Wondering each day what's the best plan for you

Thank you for the gift of seeing you just be

It's a reminder that there is a power greater than me

That I get to live my dream

Babies in plastic boxes they're my favorite team

Thank you, little fighter, you're my inspiration

I hope to see you at my next station

Keep flying, little one

For to me, your light is like sun

By Dr. Terri MD, The Preemie Doc

Reference List Entries

Altman, Lawrence. 2013. "A Kennedy Baby's Life and Death." *New York Times*, July 29, 2013. https://www.ny-times.com/2013/07/30/health/a-kennedy-babys-life-and-death.html

Blakemore, Erin. 2018. "Baby Incubators: From Board-walk Sideshow to Medical Marvel." September 12, 2018. https://www.history.com/news/baby-incubators-board-walk-sideshows-medical-marvels

Campbell-Yeo, Marsha, Disher, Timothy, Benoit, Britney, and Johnston, C Celeste. 2015. "Understanding Kangaroo Care and its Benefits to Preterm Infants." *Pediatric Health, Medicine, and Therapeutics* 16: 15-32. March 18, 2015. https://www.ncbi.nlm.nih.gov/pmc/articles/PMC568 3265/

Fagan, Abigail. 2010. "Touching Empathy." March 1, 2010. https://www.psychologytoday.com/us/blog/born-love/201003/touching-empathy

History.com Editors, 2021. "Susan Smith Reports a False Carjacking to Cover Her Murder." Published November 13, 2009. Updated October 26, 2021. https://www.history.com/this-day-in-history/susan-smith-reports-a-false-carjacking-to-cover-her-murder

Keeling, Arlene. 2015. "Historical Perspectives on an Expanded Role for Nursing." *OJIN: The Online Journal of Issues in Nursing* 20 no. 2, manuscript 2. May 31, 2015. https://ojin.nursingworld.org/MainMenuCategories/ANAMarketplace/ANAPeriodicals/OJIN/TableofContents/Vol-20-2015/No2-May-2015/Historical-Perspectives-Expanded-Role-Nursing.html

Moon, Rachel, Tanabe, Kawai, Choi Yang, Diane, Young, Heather, and Hauck, Fern. 2012. "Pacifier Use and SIDS: Evidence for a Consistently Reduced Risk." *Matern Child Health* 16 no. 3: 609-614. April 2012. https://pubmed.ncbi.nlm.nih.gov/21505778/

About the Author

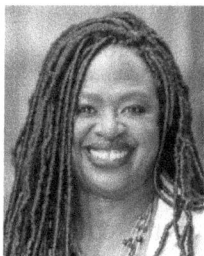

Dr. Terri Lynn Major-Kincade is a double board-certified neonatologist and pediatrician who gained national recognition through appearances on the ABC television documentary *Houston Medical* and the Lifetime Channel series *Women Docs*. She earned her bachelor of science from Prairie View A&M University, master in public health and doctor of medicine from UCLA, and a certificate in palliative care education and practice from Harvard. She completed her pediatric residency training at UT Southwestern Medical Center-Children's Medical Center Dallas and her neonatal-perinatal training at UT Houston Health Science Center-Memorial Hermann Children's Hospital. Bestselling author and renowned keynote speaker, Dr. Terri serves on numerous professional advisory boards, including Pampers Womb to World and the nonprofits Texas March of Dimes, Return to Zero HOPE, and Pregnancy Loss and Infant Death Alliance.

With a passion for empowering families to make informed choices for their babies, Dr. Terri is cherished for her authenticity and empathy in discussing challenging topics, including health equity, racial health disparities, and neonatal palliative care. She has been happily married for over twenty-five years and lives in Dallas, Texas, with her husband and two children.

Learn more at www.drterrimd.com

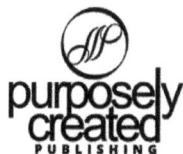

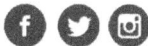

www.ingramcontent.com/pod-product-compliance
Lightning Source LLC
Chambersburg PA
CBHW071700210326
41597CB00017B/2259